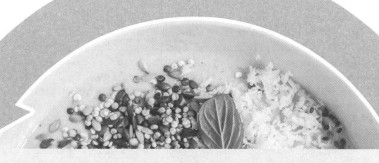

PREDIABETES:
A COMPLETE GUIDE

Your Lifestyle Reset to Stop Prediabetes and Other Chronic Illnesses

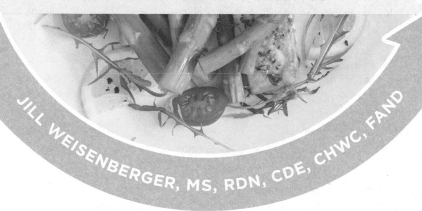

JILL WEISENBERGER, MS, RDN, CDE, CHWC, FAND

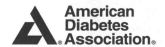

American
Diabetes
Association.

Associate Publisher, Books, Abe Ogden; *Director, Book Operations,* Victor Van Beuren; *Associate Director, Book Marketing,* Katie Curran; *Senior Manager, Book Editing,* Lauren Wilson; *Project Manager,* Wendy Martin-Shuma; *Composition,* Circle Graphics; *Cover Design,* Vis-a-vis Creative; *Illustrations,* Circle Graphics; *Printer,* Versa Press.

Printed in the United States of America
3 5 7 9 10 8 6 4

The suggestions and information contained in this publication are generally consistent with the Standards of Medical Care in Diabetes and other policies of the American Diabetes Association, but they do not represent the policy or position of the Association or any of its boards or committees. Reasonable steps have been taken to ensure the accuracy of the information presented. However, the American Diabetes Association cannot ensure the safety or efficacy of any product or service described in this publication. Individuals are advised to consult a physician or other appropriate health care professional before undertaking any diet or exercise program or taking any medication referred to in this publication. Professionals must use and apply their own professional judgment, experience, and training and should not rely solely on the information contained in this publication before prescribing any diet, exercise, or medication. The American Diabetes Association—its officers, directors, employees, volunteers, and members—assumes no responsibility or liability for personal or other injury, loss, or damage that may result from the suggestions or information in this publication.

Erika Gebel Berg conducted the internal review of this book to ensure that it meets American Diabetes Association guidelines.

⊚ The paper in this publication meets the requirements of the ANSI Standard Z39.48-1992 (permanence of paper).

ADA titles may be purchased for business or promotional use or for special sales. To purchase more than 50 copies of this book at a discount, or for custom editions of this book with your logo, contact the American Diabetes Association at the address below or at booksales@diabetes.org.

American Diabetes Association
2451 Crystal Drive, Suite 900
Arlington, VA 22202

DOI: 10.2337/9781580406741

Library of Congress Cataloging-in-Publication Data

Names: Weisenberger, Jill, author.
Title: Prediabetes : a complete guide : your lifestyle reset to stop
   prediabetes and other chronic illnesses / Jill Weisenberger MS, RDN, CDE,
   CHWC, FAND.
Description: Arlington : American Diabetes Association, [2018] | Includes
   bibliographical references and index.
Identifiers: LCCN 2017058162 | ISBN 9781580406741
Subjects: LCSH: Prediabetic state--Popular works. |
   Diabetes--Prevention--Popular works.
Classification: LCC RC660.4 .W453 2018 | DDC 616.4/6205--dc23
LC record available at https://lccn.loc.gov/2017058162

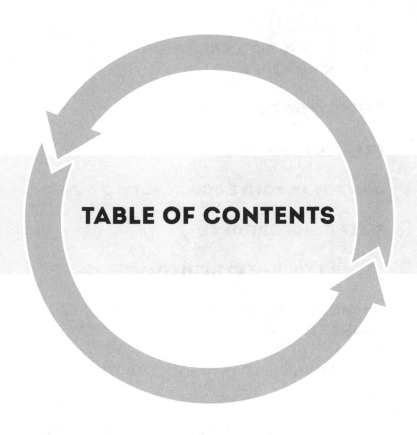

TABLE OF CONTENTS

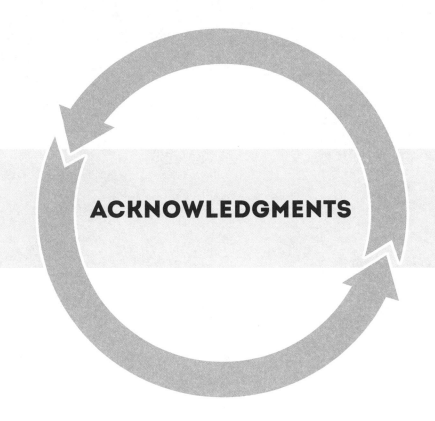

ACKNOWLEDGMENTS

My heartfelt thanks go to all those who supported me in bringing this book from idea to reality. So many people at the American Diabetes Association—many who I call my friends and some whom I've never met in person—have expertly guided me, helped me flesh out ideas, and fixed my mistakes. They have edited, illustrated, and designed this book with such care and skill that I am hugely grateful and quite proud of the finished product. My patients and clients are the ones who continue to inspire me. Thank you for sharing your stories and allowing me glimpses into your lives. There isn't a way to thank my family enough. They ground me, support me, keep me sane, entertain me, and love me no matter what project has my attention. Thank you for all you do and all that you are.

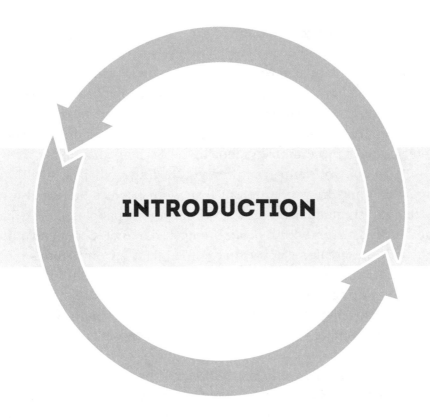

INTRODUCTION

There are many ways to a healthy plate and a healthy body. And there are many scientifically sound diet and lifestyle strategies to help you prevent type 2 diabetes, as well as medical strategies such as taking the medication metformin. However, it seems that quite a number of people continue to look for that one *best* diet. Some will flit from diet plan to diet plan in search for the one that sheds pounds, whittles the waist, boosts energy, and drives blood glucose and cholesterol levels down. Then sooner or later, something in the plan becomes unsustainable—it's boring, expensive, or overly restrictive—and the search for the best diet continues.

Success in meeting health goals doesn't start with identifying the best diet or a top-10 foods list. Rather it comes from identifying *your* best diet and *your* best healthful lifestyle habits. If I gave you advice that simply didn't fit with your life or food preferences, it wouldn't help you meet your goals no matter how strong the evidence for my advice. Fortunately, there's more than one smart way to reach your goal! Similarly, many people ask for written meal plans, but my experience tells me that they rarely help the way people expect them to. That's because most people need more flexibility than prewritten meal plans offer. Instead of meal plans, you'll find meal-planning tools and strategies and a few example menus in the chapters that follow.

This book will help empower you to find your best healthful way, which may be very different from your friend's preferred way to achieve a similar outcome. For example, many people manage diabetes or prediabetes with a vegan or vegetarian diet. Others do quite well with the greater variety that comes with an omnivore's diet. Some people meet their exercise goals and achieve cardiovascular fitness by hitting the gym several days per week. Others enjoy the solitude of jogging in their neighborhoods and strength training at home. While others join tennis, bowling, or soccer leagues to boost their fitness.

Throughout this book, you will learn about general guidelines and recommendations for good health and diabetes prevention that are grounded in science. You have the flexibility to pick a path that suits you. Simply speaking, after examining where you are in your habits today and comparing them to where you want to be eventually, you'll select small steps that lead you in that direction. And then you'll take on more and more small steps. The informational sections, exercises, worksheets, and goal-setting strategies in this book will guide you in much the same ways that I coach and counsel my clients. For accountability and expert feedback, you may want to work with a registered dietitian nutritionist (RD or RDN) who has a background in prediabetes, diabetes, and heart health.

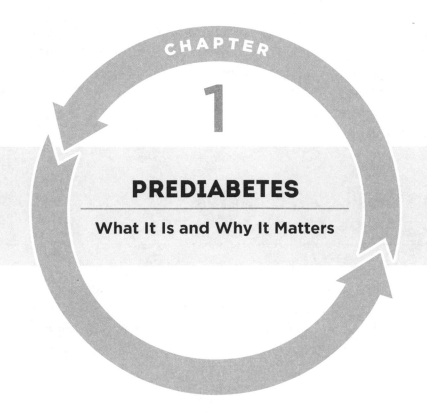

CHAPTER

1

PREDIABETES

What It Is and Why It Matters

*P*rediabetes, the leading risk factor for type 2 diabetes, is a wake-up call. The condition, which afflicts approximately 84 million American adults, is a sign that something is metabolically awry. Unfortunately, only about 12% of people with prediabetes are aware that they have this problem. Although it sounds scary to have a metabolic disorder, there is so much you can do to prevent it from getting worse. In fact, many people who improve their lifestyle habits (some take medicine, too) are able to do more than prevent type 2 diabetes; some are even able to reverse prediabetes. Without changes, however, 37% of individuals with prediabetes are likely to progress to full-blown type 2 diabetes within 4 years, and most will have the diagnosis within 10 years. Many will develop heart disease as well, even if they don't move on to diabetes. Even some types of cancers are linked to prediabetes and type 2 diabetes. Because we don't really feel prediabetes and there are often no symptoms, it's easy to ignore it and to put off making changes. Don't be tempted by that. You'll see why in the next sections. Keep reminding yourself that this is an opportunity to reverse the course. There's really quite a lot to celebrate!

Diagnosing Prediabetes and Diabetes

You have prediabetes if your blood glucose level is higher than normal, but below the level of diabetes. The chart below shows you the tests and results that health care providers use to diagnose diabetes and prediabetes. If you have an abnormal result, your health care provider will order a second test to confirm your diagnosis.

Blood Glucose Levels to Diagnose Prediabetes and Diabetes

Test	Prediabetes	Diabetes
Fasting plasma glucose	100–125 mg/dL	≥126 mg/dL
2-hour oral glucose tolerance test (OGTT)	140–199 mg/dL	≥200 mg/dL
Random plasma glucose in an individual with symptoms of diabetes such as excessive thirst and urination	Not done to diagnose prediabetes	≥200 mg/dL
A1C	5.7–6.4%	≥6.5%

What Is Borderline Diabetes?

To some people, borderline diabetes means prediabetes. To others, it means type 2 diabetes that is managed without medications. Because of the confusion, it is best to avoid using the term "borderline diabetes." If someone tells you that you have borderline diabetes, ask for clarification.

Prediabetes and Diabetes Glossary

Here are a few bits of medical jargon that you may hear when you visit your health care provider or see on your office paperwork.

A1C

A1C, also called hemoglobin A1C, is an indicator of your average blood glucose level over the past 3 months. A1C is a measure of the amount of hemoglobin within your blood cells that is coated with glucose. Hemoglobin is a protein that travels with your blood cells to provide oxygen to your tissues. If you have high levels of glucose in your blood, more glucose will stick to the hemoglobin molecule, and your A1C will be elevated. An A1C measurement between 5.7% and 6.4% is suggestive of prediabetes. If a second measurement falls within the same range, you meet the criteria for the diagnosis of prediabetes.

Impaired fasting glucose (IFG)

When your fasting blood glucose falls between 100 and 125 mg/dL, you have impaired fasting glucose. If this level is confirmed on a repeat test, you meet the criteria for the diagnosis of prediabetes.

Impaired glucose tolerance (IGT)

When the result of your 2-hour oral glucose tolerance test (OGTT) falls between 140 and 199 mg/dL, it indicates that you have impaired glucose tolerance. If this level is confirmed on a repeat test, you meet the criteria for the diagnosis of prediabetes.

Some people with prediabetes will have impaired fasting glucose. Others will have impaired glucose tolerance, and some will have both. A1C levels are affected by either or both IFG and IGT. Any two measurements (A1C, IFG, and/or IGT) can be used to diagnose prediabetes.

Type 1 diabetes

Type 1 diabetes is an autoimmune disease and affects 5–10% of Americans with diabetes. In type 1 diabetes, the pancreas is damaged because of the autoimmune dysfunction, and it makes very little insulin or no insulin at all. People with type 1 diabetes require insulin by injection or an insulin pump. Although type 1 diabetes is typically diagnosed in children and young adults, it can be diagnosed well into adulthood. Prediabetes is a risk factor for type 2 diabetes. This book is a guide to help prevent or delay type 2 diabetes only.

Blood Sugar versus Blood Glucose

"Blood sugar" and "blood glucose" mean exactly the same thing. "Blood glucose" is used throughout this book, but "blood sugar" is also commonly used in diabetes practices. Both terms refer to the concentration of glucose in the bloodstream. In the U.S., we use the unit mg/dL (milligrams glucose per deciliter of blood) to report blood glucose levels. In other parts of the world, blood glucose is reported in mmol/L (millimoles of glucose per liter of blood).

Risk Factors for Prediabetes and Type 2 Diabetes

Having prediabetes is a strong risk factor for developing type 2 diabetes. Each of the other following factors increases your risk for both prediabetes and type 2 diabetes.

Risk factors beyond your control

- Age: With each birthday, your risk grows. Health care providers usually start screening their healthy patients at age 45 years.
- Sex: Men have a greater risk than women.
- Race/ethnicity: Your risk is higher than average if you are African American, Latino, Native American, Asian American, or Pacific Islander.
- Family history: If individuals in your immediate family have prediabetes or type 2 diabetes, your risk is increased.
- Gestational diabetes: If you are a woman who previously had gestational diabetes (diabetes that occurred during pregnancy), your risk is higher.
- Polycystic ovary syndrome: If you are a woman with polycystic ovary syndrome, you have a higher chance of having prediabetes.

Take Control of These Risk Factors

Here is where you can influence your risk for developing type 2 diabetes and even reverse prediabetes. These risk factors are discussed in greater detail in later chapters. Some are directly related to the development of prediabetes and type 2 diabetes. Others may simply be signals that your risk is higher than average.

- Overweight and obesity: As weight increases, so does your risk.
- Inactivity: Being physically active helps your body use glucose better.
- High blood pressure
- High triglyceride levels
- Low HDL (good) cholesterol levels
- Heart disease or blood vessel problems
- Sleep deprivation: Too little sleep can make your body more resistant to the effects of insulin. Getting between 7 and 8 hours of sleep most nights is associated with the lowest risk of developing type 2 diabetes.
- Smoking

You can get an estimate of your risk for developing type 2 diabetes, heart disease, and stroke within the next 8 years. Simply visit the American Diabetes Association website (diabetes.org) to take the online health assessment. Click on "Are You at Risk?" on the homepage and then "My Health Advisor." This assessment is free and powerful.

Are Obesity, Prediabetes, and Type 2 Diabetes Lifestyle Diseases?

Some people feel guilty or ridiculed when they hear that the problem they have is a lifestyle disease. I can see why. Calling these problems lifestyle diseases can be interpreted as suggesting that you have caused your own illness. Even though lifestyle and behavior are critical components, they certainly aren't the only factors involved. Many people manage their weight well, eat wholesome diets, lead physically active lives, and still develop prediabetes and type 2 diabetes. Genetic and environmental factors are at play. These factors affect an individual's weight as well. In fact, the Obesity Society has identified a long list of potential contributors to overweight and obesity that boost the risk for prediabetes and type 2 diabetes. They include medications, intestinal bacteria, medical conditions, and even being born by C-section. When you hear these conditions being called lifestyle diseases, don't focus on the past. Instead, be a forward-thinker and focus on the contribution healthful lifestyle changes can make in your future. I prefer to say that these conditions have lifestyle solutions and management strategies instead of saying that they are lifestyle diseases.

Insulin Resistance and Loss of Insulin Production: Hallmarks of Prediabetes and Type 2 Diabetes

Although they often seem to, prediabetes and type 2 diabetes do not come out of the blue. Before developing type 2 diabetes, most people have prediabetes. And before they develop prediabetes, most people have insulin resistance and/or decreased insulin production with normal blood glucose levels. Unfortunately, for many, the first indicator that something is awry is some type of diabetes complication, for example, nerve pain or eye problems. Developing complications suggests that insulin resistance and decreased insulin production began many years earlier.

Type 2 diabetes, prediabetes, and insulin resistance are part of the same problem with varying levels of blood glucose. Typically, insulin resistance goes unnoticed for years because there are usually no symptoms and because blood glucose levels remain in the healthy range. Under normal circumstances, when glucose from your food enters the bloodstream, the β-cells of your pancreas send out insulin to usher excess glucose from the blood into various cells of the body. Insulin also tells the liver to stop releasing glucose excessively. Once inside these cells, glucose is either used for energy or stored for later use. But in the presence of insulin resistance, the cells of the liver, fat, muscle, and other organs become stubborn and do not react properly to the effects of insulin. When this happens, you have lost insulin sensitivity or have become insulin resistant. Blood glucose levels rise because of the progressive loss of insulin production in the presence of insulin resistance.

Here is the usual progression to type 2 diabetes.

1. *β-Cell dysfunction often alongside insulin resistance with normal blood glucose levels.* Genetics plays a big role in the development of type 2 diabetes; some people have genes that predispose the β-cells to break down. This predisposition increases the risk for the development of diabetes, especially in people whose cells become resistant to the effects of insulin. This resistance to insulin requires the β-cells of the pancreas to send out extra insulin to move glucose out of the blood and into the cells. The result is higher-than-normal insulin levels with normal blood glucose levels.

2. *Prediabetes.* The β-cells of the pancreas stop releasing enough insulin to maintain normal blood glucose levels. Blood glucose

levels rise slightly even though insulin levels are likely still higher than normal.

3. *Type 2 diabetes.* The β-cells fail even more, and the pancreas is unable to keep up with the demands. There isn't enough insulin available to keep blood glucose levels down, so they rise even higher.

Insulin Resistance Affects More than Blood Glucose Levels

Although insulin is best known for its role in controlling blood glucose levels, it actually has many roles in the body. Although cause and effect are uncertain, insulin resistance, high levels of insulin in the blood, and insufficient insulin production are often associated with other health problems, including these:

- Fatty liver
- Blood vessel dysfunction
- High blood pressure
- Low HDL (good) cholesterol levels
- Elevated triglyceride levels
- Chronic inflammation
- Increased blood clotting

These factors and others put people with prediabetes and diabetes at a higher risk of developing heart disease and having a heart attack. Thus, there's more reason to focus on lifestyle solutions. Fortunately, the steps you take to prevent type 2 diabetes do double and triple work by helping with other health concerns.

Lifestyle Interventions to Prevent Diabetes

So far, we've covered statistics and health risks, but here starts the good news. From the foods you eat to the walks you take and perhaps even the hours you sleep and more, your lifestyle habits affect your well-being and the likelihood that you will avoid or slow down the transition to type 2 diabetes. It is much easier to reverse or halt the progression of prediabetes than it is to reverse or halt the progression of type 2 diabetes. If you've been diagnosed with prediabetes or have been told that you're at high risk for developing type 2 diabetes, you have an opportunity to grab control of your health right now and be in greater charge of your future. Considering the scores of people with undiagnosed prediabetes, you are lucky to know about your risks. The best time to start making changes you can live with is right now! Because this problem is progressive, every day, the window of opportunity closes ever so slightly. Tomorrow is a good time, too, but today is even better. Your actions can boost insulin sensitivity and protect your insulin-producing β-cells.

Research proves lifestyle changes to be a winning strategy. The federally funded Diabetes Prevention Program (DPP) included more than 3,000 overweight people at risk for type 2 diabetes. Individuals who were enrolled in the intensive lifestyle change group reduced their risk of developing type 2 diabetes by 58% during the 3-year study. Even 10 years after the start of the study, the lifestyle interventions lowered the risk by 34%. And 15 years after the study started, the risk was still 27% lower.

And there was a bonus for the heart. Years after the start of the DPP, individuals in the lifestyle change group had better cholesterol and triglyceride levels and healthier blood pressure, even though they took fewer medications for these conditions. Plus, they showed less evidence of chronic inflammation.

Before the DPP was the Finnish Diabetes Prevention Study. Researchers in this study also found remarkable results. After only 2 years, the incidence of diabetes in the intervention group was less than half of what it was in the group who did not receive diet and lifestyle training. Not surprisingly, individuals who made the most dietary changes and lost the most weight had the greatest results.

So now you see you are in the driver's seat. No matter where you are starting today, you can influence your future health.

Winning Strategies of the Diabetes Prevention Program

The aim of the lifestyle change group of the DPP was to help participants to lose 7% of their body weight (14 pounds for someone starting at 200 pounds) and to engage in 150 minutes of physical activity each week. Additionally, program facilitators guided participants to do the following:

- Monitor their weight regularly
- Keep track of their physical activity
- Reduce their calorie intake
- Eat a wholesome, balanced diet
- Record their food intake
- Manage stress
- Focus on stopping unhelpful negative thoughts
- Develop problem-solving skills related to healthful eating and being active
- Maintain motivation

The original program also encouraged a reduced-fat diet. That aspect is no longer part of ongoing diabetes prevention programs. Newer science tells us that the quality of the fat is far more important than the quantity of fat that we consume. Today, scientists and health care professionals encourage wholesome foods with unsaturated fat such as avocados, nuts, salmon, and liquid oils and discourage foods rich in unhealthful saturated and trans fats (see Chapter 3 for more on fats).

Metabolic Syndrome: A Related Disorder

Metabolic syndrome describes a group of risk factors for developing type 2 diabetes, heart disease, and stroke. What this underscores is that these three common health problems are related. Look at the list of five metabolic risk factors below. A person with three or more risk factors has metabolic syndrome and is at high risk for developing type 2 diabetes, heart disease, and stroke. If you research the metabolic syndrome, you may see slightly different numbers. Various organizations define metabolic syndrome differently, and there are different numbers for different ethnic groups.

1. Elevated triglyceride levels: ≥150 mg/dL or taking medication for high triglyceride levels
2. Low HDL cholesterol levels: <40 mg/dL in men and <50 mg/dL in women or taking medication to treat low HDL cholesterol levels
3. High blood pressure: top number (systolic blood pressure) ≥130 mmHg or bottom number (diastolic blood pressure) ≥85 mmHg or taking medication to treat high blood pressure
4. Elevated fasting blood glucose: ≥100 mg/dL or taking medication to lower blood glucose levels
5. Large waistline: ≥40 inches men and ≥35 inches in women (however, risk starts at smaller waistlines in some ethnic populations)

Boosting Insulin Sensitivity and Preserving Insulin Production

Boosting insulin sensitivity and boosting or preserving insulin production are keys to halting prediabetes. Here are four things to do just that. They are each covered in great detail in the coming chapters.

1. *Weight loss.* As seen in the DPP and other studies, losing just a little weight—not tons of weight—reverses insulin resistance and lowers the risk for developing type 2 diabetes.
2. *Diet.* Weight loss is very hard. If it weren't, there would be few overweight people. It's good news that even without weight

loss, a healthful diet can help you. The American Diabetes Association notes that diets with higher intakes of nuts, berries, yogurt, coffee, and tea are associated with less risk of diabetes. Red meats and sugar-sweetened beverages are associated with an increased risk of developing the disease. There are many tips on having a healthful diet throughout this book and in Chapter 3.

3. *Physical activity.* It's too bad that so many people focus on the weight loss benefits of exercise because exercise does so much more than that. Every single time you exercise, you boost insulin sensitivity. Every. Single. Time.

4. *Sleep.* We live in a sleep-deprived world. Unfortunately, lack of sleep hinders your body's use of insulin. As you'll see in Chapter 10, it's a good idea to aim for 7–8 hours of sleep nightly.

Medical Management of Prediabetes

Medications are another tool to help prevent type 2 diabetes. The DPP found good results with the drug metformin, a common medication used to treat type 2 diabetes. Metformin is an insulin sensitizer. It helps your body use insulin more effectively. It also lowers blood glucose levels by decreasing the amount of glucose created and released by your liver.

There were three study groups in the DPP. Some participants were enrolled in the lifestyle change group. Others joined the metformin group, and the rest made up the control group and received only basic diet and exercise information. Overall metformin wasn't as effective as intensive lifestyle modification, but the results were still worth celebrating. In the 3 years of the DPP, metformin reduced the risk of developing diabetes by 31%—a positive result, but not as impressive as the 58% reduction experienced by individuals in the lifestyle change group. After 10 years, metformin reduced the risk by 18%, and after 15 years, the drug reduced the risk by 17%. Intensive lifestyle changes still brought about more positive change, but metformin created impressive results as well, particularly among specific groups of people.

Because of the results of the DPP, the American Diabetes Association recommends that metformin therapy be considered for people who are very obese, individuals younger than 60 years, women who previously had gestational diabetes, and individuals who have A1C levels ≥6%.

Your health care provider may prescribe metformin along with lifestyle changes. Also, as research continues to find additional medications to halt the progression of prediabetes to type 2 diabetes, you may be prescribed a different medication.

Treatment for Related Obesity and Cardiovascular Risk Factors

Because weight loss is an important prevention strategy, you and your health care provider may discuss the medical management of weight loss, too. There are now several weight loss medications used in conjunction with lifestyle changes that help people lose 5–10% of their starting weight and sometimes even more. Weight loss surgery is another avenue to weight loss. Depending on the type of surgery, people lose on average 15% of their starting weight up to about one-third of their starting weight.

Finally, because both prediabetes and diabetes are linked to higher rates of heart disease, you and your health care provider must also address your blood pressure and cholesterol levels. Medications may be in order for these cardiovascular risk factors. The truly good news here is that the lifestyle changes that help prevent type 2 diabetes will also help you prevent heart disease. As new habits are formed and you become healthier, you may be able to lower the dosages of some medications or stop taking them altogether. Just don't make changes without talking it through with a member of your health care team first.

Be Empowered

Knowledge is power, but only if you also take action. Empower yourself with both information and real change.

- Review the section Risk Factors for Prediabetes and Type 2 Diabetes and try to identify your risk factors.
- Take the online diabetes risk test. Encourage your friends and family members to do the same.
- It is rare that a person with prediabetes is aware of the condition. Ask your health care provider if you should be screened for the disorder. Encourage your friends and family members to discuss it with their health care providers, too.
- If you have prediabetes or are otherwise at high risk for developing type 2 diabetes, commit some time to work through this book. You can make a difference, beginning right now, one small step at a time.
- If you'd like additional help and accountability, ask your health care provider for a referral to a registered dietitian nutritionist.
- For a different type of accountability and for empowering messages, share your progress and setbacks on social media. Use the hashtag #LifestyleReset and tag me, @NutritionJill.

2

PREPARING FOR YOUR LIFESTYLE RESET

*K*nowing what you want your health to look like and why you want to make changes are really the first steps to success. Simply stating that I want to be thinner or healthier is rarely concrete enough to keep you going when motivation wanes or strong enough to keep you focused when you're extra tired, busy, or irritated. You can boost your chances of meeting your goals by having a clear picture of what success means. Focusing on skills, strategies, and habits, instead of willpower, is an important component to long-term success. By examining your overall health goals, identifying your motivators, learning to set meaningful behavioral goals, and setting a plan to develop health-boosting habits, you up your odds of celebrating success. These are the things we begin to cover in this chapter. Please resist the temptation to skip over these sections requiring self-reflection and deep planning. I understand why you might want to—it feels weird, takes up time, seems too basic, etc. But I have known so many very motivated, very smart people fail to make long-term changes. They insisted on relying on willpower instead of creating a careful plan based on their individual lives, thought processes, and motivators. Healthful living and weight management are not about character. Mastering these areas requires having the right strategies, a positive attitude, solid skills, and a flexible plan.

Imagine Your Healthiest Self

A personal wellness vision is a concrete and motivating picture of you being healthy, feeling healthy, and living a healthful life. Imagine yourself at your ideal level of well-being. How do you feel? Look? Act? What are you doing that brings you joy and a sense of good health? It's this vision that will help you set goals—both long term and short term—and stay focused on them. Without putting in the time to create this picture of your healthiest self, you risk setting weak goals with weak motivators based on a vague sense of wellness. A clear personal wellness vision and the goals that are born from it show you your path to better health and allow you to act with intention.

Here are two examples of a personal wellness vision. After reviewing the examples and the tips to creating a vision statement, grab some paper and a pencil or sit at your computer to get started on yours. It can be a work in progress. Because we make lots of changes, I always use pencil when creating vision statements with clients. Then I ask them to rewrite it in their own words and their own handwriting or to type it up neatly. This helps the client to think about, fine-tune, and edit the statement. If you'd like, use the Healthy Me template in Appendix B on page 266 to write out your wellness vision. Keep it in a handy place, so you can refer to it often.

Two Examples of Wellness Visions

Laurie's Personal Wellness Vision

I move through my day with a sense of confidence. I sit comfortably when I cross my legs. I feel strong and fit and am active without knee pain. I play tennis with my girlfriends, and I play with enthusiasm and energy. It's fun to shop for cuter, smaller clothing, and I smile when I glimpse at my reflection. Without stressing, I regularly choose wholesome foods that I enjoy and fill me with nourishment and a sense of satisfaction. I feel positive about my health and my future. I have such energy that I spin on my heels.

Brian's Personal Wellness Vision

I am strong and confident. I am able to fix things around my house and yard, and I keep up with my children and grandchildren. I enjoy traipsing all over the amusement parks with my grandkids and especially taking them on roller coasters. I have energy and good health for the missionary work that is so important to me. Eating healthful meals and snacks is second nature. I actually look forward to my annual checkup because I've tended to my cholesterol and blood glucose levels.

Tips for Creating a Personal Wellness Vision

Some people resist creating a personal wellness vision because it feels awkward or silly. And some people have a hard time putting their vision into words. Don't let these things prevent you from turning your vague ideas of what you want into a clear picture of what you're working toward. The following tips will help you create a compelling vision of your future healthy self.

- Write your statement in the present tense to make it more real and meaningful.
- Keep it positive, which is more powerful than a list of don'ts. Instead of writing about what you don't want, write about what you do want. For example, turn "I'm not winded when I walk or uncomfortable when I cross my legs," into "I walk with ease and am comfortable when I sit with my legs crossed."
- Set aside some quiet time to ask yourself what's important and why. These questions might help you.
  - What does my ideal health and fitness look like in 1, 3, and 5 years?
  - What activities am I happily participating in 1, 3, and 5 years from now?
  - How do I look then? What am I wearing then?
  - What about these things makes me happy and energized?
  - What worries have I tossed aside?
  - What are 5–10 benefits I'll get by improving my lifestyle?
  - What are at least three things that I highly value? How is my health linked to these values? For example, if you value spending time with your children or volunteering in your community, you'll need good health to be physically active and to feel energized.
  - What would my life be like if I achieved my ideal level of wellness? What would it be like if I stayed the same?

- Don't hesitate to talk to a friend or family member about this to help you see the bigger picture. Often other people know just the questions to ask. In fact, consider inviting someone close to you to also create a personal wellness vision.
- Revisit your wellness vision often. Look to it for motivation and a reminder of what you are working so hard to achieve. And feel free to tweak or change it as you learn more about yourself and your goals.

Goal-Setting

Your personal wellness vision is a picture of where you're going. Your long- and short-term behavioral goals are the blueprint to get there. I suggest that you create at least 3-month behavioral goals and weekly or other immediate goals. Three months (or even four, if you prefer) is a good amount of time to establish new routines, but not so far in the future that you can easily dismiss any sense of urgency or commitment.

3-Month Behavioral Goals

Ask yourself what habits or routines you'd like to have in place approximately 3 months from now. These behaviors should be the ones that direct you to fulfilling your personal wellness vision. To help Laurie reach her ideal level of health, she might have the following 3-month goals. Take notice of how they support her wellness vision described above. Write your own in your journal, or use the My 3-Month Behavioral Goals sheet on page 267 in Appendix B.

1. I exercise at the gym or otherwise participate in purposeful exercise at least four times each week and for a total of at least 200 minutes weekly.
2. Instead of visiting the office kitchen for a snack, I choose my afternoon snack from nourishing foods that I bring with me.

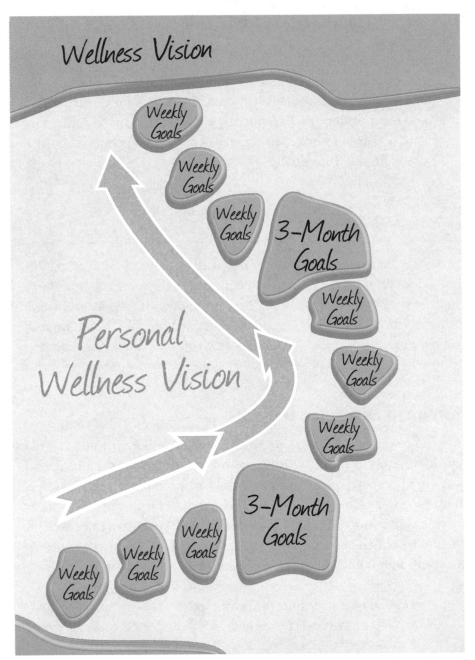

Notice how your weekly goals step you toward your 3-month goals and eventually take you all the way to your ideal vision of your wellness.

3. I pack my lunch every workday.
4. I cook dinner most nights from a selection of healthful recipes.
5. I have a regular bedtime.

Every 3 months, create a new set of 3-month behavioral goals.

Very-Short-Term Behavioral Goals

Setting 1- or 2-week goals is key to progress. These goals are small, manageable steps toward meeting your 3-month goals. Pick at least two small goals. As many as three to five is often ideal, although you should pick the number of goals that is best for you. Your goals should stretch you enough that you have to work at them and be important enough to keep you motivated and on target to your 3-month goals. But they should not be so hard that you set yourself up for failure. You do not have to address each of your 3-month goals every week. It's reasonable to work on just a couple things each week or every 2 weeks. Write your very-short-term goals on the Goal-Tracker on page 269 in Appendix B.

Think of these goals as mini experiments. You are not stuck with them beyond a week or so. One purpose of these mini experiments is to learn what you like, what you don't like, and what you are capable of doing. View these experiments with a scientist's eye. Simply observe what happens and how you feel about it. Scientists are looking for data, not judging the data. When your 1- or 2-week experiment is over, use the information you gathered to help you get closer to your 3-month goals.

Laurie might create the following weekly goals to support her 3-month goals.

1. This week, I will renew my membership at the gym.
2. At least three mornings before work this week, I will walk around my neighborhood for 10–20 minutes or engage in other purposeful exercise for the same amount of time.

3. On Monday, I'll take five pieces of fruit to work, one for each afternoon snack.

4. When I do my shopping on Saturday, I'll buy a new lunchbox and a blue-ice pack to keep my food cold.

5. This week, I'll collect at least five recipes to try and will prepare at least one of them. I'll keep my new recipes in a binder with notes about what my family likes and dislikes.

You can see that these goals are all very specific behaviors. They are not vague like the statements "to eat better" or "to exercise more," and they are not outcomes of behaviors, such as having lower blood glucose numbers or losing 2 pounds. Putting the emphasis on behaviors is really the only place you have control. You are fully in charge of your actions, but not really in charge of your body, which may sometimes seem to have a mind of its own.

Effective Goals Are SMART

- **S: Specific (or Stranger Test):** Be very clear about what you will do, how you will do it, and where you will do it. Give your goal the stranger test: If your goal is specific enough, even a stranger who reads it will know what you plan to do.
- **M: Measurable:** Can you measure your success? You should be able to recognize if you were 100% successful or 80% successful. "Eating better" and "snacking less" are not fully measurable. Rewrite your goal if it can't be objectively measured.
- **A: Action-Oriented:** Make sure that your goal is written as a behavior. What action will you take? Remember that you have control over your actions, but your body can be a bit stubborn.
- **R: Realistic:** Ask yourself if your goal is attainable with reasonable effort. Can you achieve this with the resources you

have? You should have to work at achieving your goal, but not struggle so much that you are doomed to fail.

- **T: Timely:** Know when you will do this and when you will assess the outcomes.

It is possible to be too specific or too time-bound. For example, you might say that you will walk on the beach after breakfast every day this week. That's a terrific goal unless the weather turns bad or if you have an early-morning appointment. It's a good idea to include a backup to a goal like this. In Laurie's example above, she includes the option to do other exercise if she can't or doesn't walk outside before work.

The Goal Needs a Plan

There's still more prepping to do once your goals are clearly written. You will need to look them over to see what stands in your way of success. Do you need new shoes before you walk? If you plan to eat fruit for snacks, when will you shop for them? One nice thing about setting 1- or 2-week goals is that you will quickly get very good at writing them and seeing how to make yourself successful. In Laurie's example above, she immediately realized that to pack her lunch, she needed to buy supplies. She even created a goal around that. You will find a SMART Goals Worksheet in Appendix B on page 268.

Assess Your Readiness to Work on Your Goal

You have a carefully crafted SMART goal and a plan, but are you really ready to move forward? Are you confident that you can be reasonably successful? Are you motivated and willing to put in the time and effort? Do you believe that this goal will take you closer to your wellness vision? Success is more attainable if you believe that your goal is important. If you see no value in eating breakfast, for example, eating breakfast daily is probably not a good goal for you—at least not now. Be sure to choose goals that are important to you, not goals that someone else told you were important. Likewise, it's good to be motivated to work on your goal and to be confident that you can be successful. Use the rulers below to answer each of the three questions.

1. On a scale of 1 to 10, how important is this goal to me?
2. On a scale of 1 to 10, how motivated am I to work on this goal?
3. One a scale of 1 to 10, how confident am I that with the resources I have available, I can be reasonably successful with this goal?

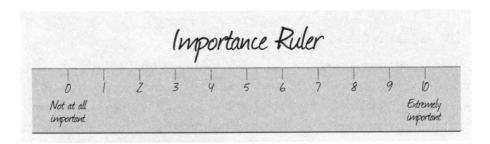

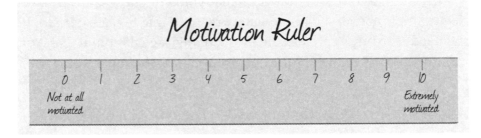

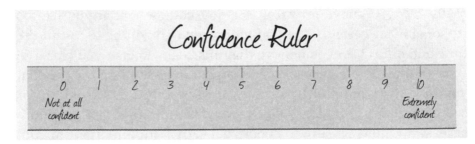

If you have identified at least a 7 on these rulers for each of the three questions, you have a good chance of being able to brag about your success. However, if you give your goal a low level of importance, say a 5 or less, you may want to hold this goal for now and work on something more relevant to you. If your motivation is high (7 or higher) but your confidence is low, ask yourself if the goal is too big or if you can do something or get some help to make success more likely.

Here's an example. Consider a goal to pack your lunch for work all 5 days next week. You've ranked it a 10 for importance, 9 for motivation, but only 5 for confidence. Carefully think about this ranking. What made you score it a 5 and not much lower, like a 2? What gives you at least a moderate level of confidence? Then explore why your confidence isn't higher and how you can boost it. Does changing your goal to pack your lunch four times next week boost your confidence? Does planning to grocery shop on the weekends lift it high enough? What about packing meals for 2 days at a time? Keep offering up new ideas to yourself until you can answer all three questions with a 7 or higher. Success brings about more success, so start wherever you are. Show yourself that you are successful.

Tracking Your Goals and Progress

Monitoring your progress is one more step to success. It's a good idea to track both your behavioral goals and their outcomes. So if weight is important to you, step on the scale regularly. If your blood glucose concerns you, ask your health care provider to share your A1C or fasting blood glucose results every 6 months or so. Or ask if you should monitor your blood glucose at home.

Keep track of your behavior-change progress with a simple Goal-Tracker like this one. Use the template on page 269 in Appendix B or create one in your journal or on your computer. Another option is to use a smartphone app.

GOAL	Day 1 Mon	Day 2 Tues	Day 3 Wed	Day 4 Thurs	Day 5 Fri	Day 6 Sat	Day 7 Sun	RESULT
I will eat breakfast every day this week.	Yes	Yes	Yes	Yes	Yes	Yes	Yes	7 of 7 times (100%)
I will take my lunch to work Monday through Thursday.	No	Yes	Yes	Yes	NA	NA	NA	3 of 4 times (75%)
I will start getting ready for bed by 10:00 each night Sunday through Thursday.	Yes	Yes	No 10:25	Yes	NA	NA	No 10:30	3 of 5 times (60%)
I will engage in purposeful exercise at least 5 days this week and for a minimum of 30 minutes each time.	30 minutes walking	35 minutes walking	40 minutes walking	10 minutes walking, 25 minutes weight training	40 minutes walking	10 minutes walking, 30 minutes weight training	35 minutes biking	7 times (>100%)

The final step in goal-setting is to assess your success. Ask your-self what you liked about working on each goal. What didn't you like? Was something surprising? What do you want to keep, toss out, or modify? How can you make your success greater and the process more fun or rewarding? These are the types of questions that will help you develop your next set of 1- or 2-week goals.

Nine Steps in the Goal-Setting Process

This summary should help you get and stay organized with this process.

1. Set a SMART goal.
2. Plan how you will implement your goal. List all the steps it will take to be successful.

3. Use the Importance Ruler to be certain this goal is truly important to you (>7).
4. Use the Motivation Ruler to assess your motivation to carry out this goal (>7).
5. Use the Confidence Ruler to assess your confidence of success with this goal (>7).
6. Rewrite your goal if necessary based on any of the above.
7. Track your progress.
8. Assess your success.
9. Plan your next goal based on this experience.

The Mighty Habit

When we talk about a lifestyle reset, we are really talking about forming new, health-boosting habits and nixing bad ones. Habits can make our lives much easier. They free up the brain to work on complex problems or unique immediate needs. Or they simply give the brain some rest.

I remember first learning to drive. When starting the car, I concentrated very hard on where my feet were and the necessary steps to back out of the garage. Use the brake, not the gas. Check the mirrors. Turn the engine on. Don't turn the ignition too far. Put the car in reverse. Check the mirrors. Lift foot off the brake. It was mentally taxing actually. Today, I sit in the car and go. I still do all of those same steps, but I hardly think of them because they are habitual. We can say the same thing about so many daily tasks. We don't really concentrate on putting milk back in the refrigerator once we're done with it. We don't struggle with the steps to tying our shoes. In fact, you probably habitually put your shoes on with the right foot first or second, but nearly always in the same order. And you probably tie them with the right or left tie crossed first, but again, always in the same order. How you put your shoes on and tie them is a pretty neutral habit, but being able to do it automatically frees you to think of other things while getting dressed, like remembering to grab your lunch before racing out the door, until that too becomes a habit.

Forming New Habits

You've probably heard that it takes 21 days to form a habit. Sadly, this is just a myth. Research points out that the length of time it takes to form a new habit varies significantly. In one study, it took participants between 18 and 254 days to establish a new health-related habit. The length of time depended on individual characteristics, things in the environment, and how hard the task was.

Whether you want to eat mindfully, reach for fruit for a snack, or take a walk after lunch, what may seem impossible to change, isn't impossible. Is it hard? Yes, probably. Very hard? That too. But what now takes lots of brainpower may soon use little mental energy and become so routine that you hardly recognize when you're engaged in the new behavior.

To purposefully form new habits, it helps to understand the habit loop, as described by Charles Duhigg in his fun-to-read bestseller, *The Power of Habit*. The habit loop consists of three components. First you have a *cue*, which is something to trigger the brain to act automatically. The second component is the *routine*, which could be a behavior or a thought. The final component is the *reward*, which is the immediate benefit that comes from the routine.

Create your own habit loop

You might find that you are compelled to check your email every time you see or hear that a new message has come in. Your *cue* is the sight or sound of a new message. Leaving another task to read the new email is the *routine*. Perhaps your *reward* is having a clean email box. There are many examples like this in your daily life. Do you check social media (routine) whenever you stand in line at the supermarket (cue)? Do you make a pit stop to eat sweets in the office lunchroom (routine) when you walk by (cue)? Do you routinely take a walk (routine) after you clear the dinner dishes (cue)?

Use knowledge of this habit loop to form new habits. Perhaps the easiest place to start is to pick your cue. Start with a current habit

Morning Habit Loop

Cue
Kids leave
for school

Routine
Have coffee
and pastry

Reward
Peaceful
time alone

and link another to it. One of my clients is currently working on forming the habit of exercising before work. We talked about her current morning routine and decided that she would lace up her shoes and head outside for a walk or into the living room to dance to music as soon as she put her morning coffee cup into the dishwasher, a habit already ingrained. She is attempting to link a morning walk or dance (routine) to her current behavior of putting her coffee cup away (cue).

I have successfully linked a new behavior (routine) to an existing behavior (cue) dozens of times. An example unrelated to health has to do with watering the plants on my front porch. For years, my hanging baskets and potted plants would die from neglect, until I linked watering them to a regular habit. My family has our milk delivered, so I rinse the empty bottles and leave them for our milkman. Frustrated with myself for letting our plants die, I brainstormed some ideas for a cue. This was a simple solution because I have to put the bottles outside anyway. Now I rinse them, fill them with fresh water, and give my plants a drink before putting the empty bottles in the crate for our milkman. I'm happy to report that none of my plants has withered from neglect since I started this behavior.

Don't forget to build in your reward. Sometimes the reward of exercise is the release of feel-good brain chemicals that comes during a hard workout. But sometimes the exercise was a drag, and we have to force ourselves to keep going. That's where we need to insert an obvious reward. I encourage my clients to give themselves the pat on the back they deserve. Take several seconds after you accomplish a task to fully appreciate your effort. I don't mean a 1-second, "Yay, I did it." Fully embrace the feelings of accomplishment and the effort you gave it. Feel the pride for 10 or 20 or 30 seconds. Without reward, change is hard.

Nixing Bad Habits

Perhaps you want to break the habit of automatically eating second and third helpings at dinner and grabbing a snack every time you walk by the kitchen at your home or office. Starting with the cue is often the easiest place to break an unproductive habit, too. Examine what leads you to unhealthful behaviors. What is the cue? If the cue is seeing treats in the kitchen, can you avoid the kitchen? Can you arrange that office sweets are put on a counter not seen from the doorway? One client successfully avoided the office kitchen simply by packing a thermal bottle with coffee every morning. She could still enjoy her coffee without going near tempting treats. Another client stopped nibbling on cookies at home once she decided to store them in a cabinet she rarely opened. And a few clients over the years have broken their habits of eating a donut or two on their morning commutes simply by driving a couple of blocks out of the way to avoid the donut shop flashing a "Hot Now" sign.

You might also break a bad habit by replacing it with a new one. I know lots of people, including myself, who nixed nighttime snacking by brushing their teeth immediately after dinner. We simply used the cue of getting up from the table or carrying dirty dishes to the sink as a reminder to brush our teeth. With clean teeth and a fresh mouth, it's easier to avoid recreational eating.

Look at your cue, but also look at your reward. What is the reward from sitting with a bowl of ice cream late at night? If the reward is time to yourself or something indulgent, you don't need a bowl of ice cream. You can indulge in other ways: a good book, sipping exotic tea from a fancy mug, or even by giving yourself a foot massage. The key is to do this new behavior regularly, so it becomes the replacement habit.

Guard Healthy Habits

New habits are tenuous. They can be easily broken. Even longstanding habits are fragile under certain circumstances such as moving to a new home, starting a new job, getting injured or sick, and getting married. Guard your habits fiercely. If a change in your daily schedule keeps you from attending exercise class after breakfast, spend a few minutes walking or stretching to maintain the routine of exercise after breakfast. Once you're back to your usual schedule, you'll still have the habit of morning exercise. If you have formed the habit of preparing a salad and another vegetable for supper, don't let the change of seasons ruin your healthy plate. Think through what it will take to keep your vegetable habit. Will it be making soup in the winter? Using more canned or frozen and fewer fresh vegetables? There are many possible solutions. For tips to create a structured plan, look at the HURDLE Method to Overcoming Obstacles later in this chapter.

Nine Steps to Forming a Good Habit

Using the concept of the habit loop described above, you can create purposeful new habits. These nine steps offer additional guidance and a structure you can return to often.

1. *Start small.* The key is to become consistent, so make it as easy as possible to achieve success right away. If, for example, your ultimate goal is to walk for 30 minutes every morning before work, get into the routine quickly by walking just 5 or 10 minutes every day. You're more likely to form a habit in this short daily walk than you are in a longer walk just once or twice a week. Keep in mind that success breeds more success, so starting small can lead to something big.

2. *Link your new habit to an existing one.* As discussed in greater detail above, tying the new behavior to something you're already doing is a smart way to become consistent with the desired behavior. If you want to keep a water bottle full, plan to refill it each time you get up to answer the phone. If you want to start packing your lunch, link that to cleaning up your kitchen after dinner. Think about things you do each day and things that happen each day. Some examples: Shower, brush your teeth, use the restroom, drink coffee, check the mail, check email, let the dogs out, let the dogs in, the phone rings, eat a meal, read the paper.

3. *Choose a manageable number of new habits to work on.* This will vary from person to person, but most won't work on more than four or five new habits at a time. To maximize success, it's better to aim to change fewer things. So many people are hypermotivated to achieve a rapid overhaul that they quickly become overwhelmed and lose any progress they make early on.

4. *Think convenience.* Plan to exercise or pack your lunch at times that actually fit your schedule. Beyond that, be sure that you have the necessary supplies. You'll need comfortable shoes and

socks for walking and something to carry your lunch in and keep it cold. Have these things handy. It's much harder to form a new habit if you can't find the things you need.

5. *Reward yourself.* Identify an immediate reward and focus on it. Your reward may be a sense of pride, feeling more satisfied or comfortable after a meal, having a runner's high, great taste, less afternoon fatigue, or saving a few bucks by avoiding take-out. It doesn't matter what it is, as long as it's important to you and you spend some time acknowledging it.

6. *Create an if-then statement.* This is how you safeguard your desired behavior when life gets in the way. If your goal is to walk outside before work, your *if-then* statement might look like this: If it's raining, I'll ride my stationary bike instead of walking outside. If you're working to prepare dinner most nights, you might have an *if-then* statement like this: If I get home late from after-school activities, I'll prepare a quick dinner from frozen items or pantry staples like canned tuna, whole-grain crackers, and fruit.

7. *Track it.* Create a SMART goal around your new desired behavior, and use the Goal-Tracker first described on page 28 or some other method of monitoring your behavior. One of my clients has a bulletin board–sized calendar to which she adds different color stickers for various behaviors. I've even heard of the paper clip method. With this method, a person starts the day with a certain number of paper clips and moves one to a dish or a pocket each time the behavior is performed. For example, you might start your day with a string of 10 paper clips, one for each glass of unsweetened drink you want to consume. After drinking one glass of water or unsweetened tea, move one paper clip from your string of paper clips to a dish, your pocket, or a paper clip holder. Some people prefer apps on their smartphones. Whatever you choose to use, use it consistently (yes, that's a habit, too). The act of tracking and the visual cues tracking provides reinforce your desired behavior.

8. *Assess it.* Set aside some thinking time to review your progress. Remember to view your progress without judgment. Allow the data to inform you and to help you tweak your goals or your plans.

9. *Join forces.* It helps to have a partner. Work with a friend, family member, or a professional such as a registered dietitian nutritionist (RD or RDN) or a credentialed health coach.

Nine Tips to Nixing a Bad Habit

It's hard to break into the mind when it's operating on autopilot. Thus, extinguishing a bad habit usually takes considerable effort. Sometimes it's much harder to stop a bad habit than to create a good one. Willpower is not the answer. Willpower is magical thinking. After identifying an unhelpful habit to stamp out, try these nine tips.

1. *Identify the benefit.* Even bad habits offer some benefit. Maybe spending time on social media gives you a needed break from household chores, paying bills, or working. Dinner from the drive-thru saves you time. Snacking on your commute home lessens the boredom. Try to identify each possible benefit of the bad habit. There may be many.

2. *Pick another way to achieve the same benefit.* Certainly, you can take a more productive break from work or chores such as writing in a journal or even socializing with a friend for a few minutes. There are other ways to save time in your day than to skip a wholesome meal. And listening to a podcast or recorded book makes an afternoon commute zip by. The point is to brainstorm ways to maintain a reward.

3. *Identify your cues.* What things in your environment or what thoughts trigger the undesired behavior? For some people, seeing a "Hot Now" sign triggers a craving for donuts. Seeing chocolate in the pantry might spark a taste for it. Feeling lonely or worried might summon up the desire for a favorite comfort food. Putting the kids to bed may signal it's time for dessert.

4. *Remove cues.* As I mentioned earlier, I've had a handful of donut lovers avoid the urge simply by driving a route that didn't pass a donut shop. Other people have removed trigger foods from sight. And I keep chocolate in a cabinet I rarely open for any reason other than to treat myself.

5. *Feel the urge.* Some triggers can't be removed, but we can relearn how to respond to them. Mindfulness experts teach us to explore and fully experience the urge to engage in the unwanted behavior. Some call it surfing the urge. You can minimize the power a craving or urge has over you by observing it without judgment. You will likely see that cravings don't simply get stronger, even though they sometimes feel like they will never end. Rather, they build, peak, and drop off similar to an ocean's wave. Try it. When an urge comes over you, sit quietly and watch it without battling it. Where do you feel it in your body? What do you feel? Focus on your breath. Don't argue with the urge, and don't try to beat it. Just observe it. Most likely, the urge will crash and wash away in only a few minutes. Like other new behaviors, this takes practice to perfect.

6. *Substitute a new routine.* One of my patients nixed nighttime snacking by picking up needlework. Another person gargles with a strong mouthwash after dinner. If you've accurately identified your cues or triggers, you might find success with a replacement behavior.

7. *Visualize success.* Learn to ignore your triggers by imagining yourself being successful. If you want to stop unhealthful snacking in the car, imagine getting into the driver's seat, take note that there are no snacks nearby, take satisfaction in that, and visualize yourself driving your usual route being perfectly comfortable without eating. Finally, praise your success. This step also is a strategy that takes practice, so don't get discouraged if it feels awkward at first or if you need many visualization sessions before a craving loses its power over you. Some

people visualize the desired behavior daily until they are secure in their new routine.

8. *Assess it.* Again, set aside some time to focus on your progress. Remember to view your experience with a scientist's eye. You're collecting data to help you appropriately change your plan.

9. *Join forces.* If you need more help, seek out a friend, family member, or professional.

HURDLE Method to Overcoming Obstacles

Part of forming new habits and successfully ticking behaviors on your goal sheet is anticipating obstacles and planning to overcome them. For example, how will you manage your alcohol intake at an upcoming wedding or fit in your daily exercise when you have houseguests. Eventually, looking for impediments to your success will also become second nature. For now, use this HURDLE method. The worksheet on page 270 in Appendix B will guide you through each step.

Defining HURDLE

- **H: How** is your upcoming schedule different? Think about your day and look at your calendar for appointments and activities. Is there something unusual or at an unusual time?
- **U: Understand** how these events, appointments, or obligations could derail you from your healthy lifestyle goals. Will something prevent you from eating a meal, getting to exercise class on time, or getting to bed at the usual hour? Will someone else be in charge of your meals or your schedule?
- **R: Record** your options. Brainstorm and write down every possible solution, even the silly ones.
- **D: Decide** on a solution. Pick one or more realistic options from your list of possible solutions.

- **L: List** the steps. Record everything that you must do to make this solution work. Include if you need to buy things, wake up early, change your schedule, ask for help, etc.
- **E: Exercise** your choice and **Evaluate** it. Carry out your selected option. Make notes about how it went, what you learned, and what you will do differently next time.

Here's an example of how to use the HURDLE method:

- **H: How:** Beth's parents will be visiting for a week.
- **U: Understand:** Over the last 8 months, Beth has changed her cooking and food choices to provide more wholesome food for her family. Beth and her family attempt to follow a Mediterranean-style eating pattern, rich in plant proteins, fish, whole grains, fruits, and vegetables. Beth grew up eating Southern fried chicken, biscuits, sweet tea, and other foods she now finds greasy and unhealthful. Her parents continue to eat like this, and Beth is expected to prepare meals and shop for groceries while her parents are in town. Beth worries that she'll lose health gains if she prepares the food her parents expect.
- **R: Record:** Beth jots down these options.
  - Ask her parents not to come.
  - Prepare two sets of meals.
  - Prepare the foods she usually prepares.
  - Prepare the foods she usually prepares with some modification.
  - Prepare Southern-style food in more healthful ways.
  - Ask her parents to prepare their own food if they don't like what she's cooking.
  - Eat out most nights, so everyone can order what they like.
- **D: Decide:** Beth decides to stick with her family's usual diet and make a few changes to please her parents.

- **L: List:** Beth lists these steps to her action plan.
    - Call her mom to inform her parents about the family's current diet.
    - Send her mom a list of foods Beth likes to cook now and ask her mom which foods are most likely to be accepted.
    - Plan her menus for the week to include mostly the foods her parents have given a favorable nod to. Add a few family favorites from her childhood that Beth can modify to make more wholesome.
    - Make a shopping list based on her planned menus. Add ready-to-bake biscuits and a few other foods that her parents love. Beth can add them to her otherwise Mediterranean-style meals.
    - Purchase the food.
    - Each night, prepare a wholesome meal. Two or three times out of the week, add a favorite of her parents, such as biscuits or a trimmed-down version of macaroni and cheese.
- **E: Exercise** and **Evaluate:** Beth executed her plan as expected, and she is so pleased with the outcome. Her parents accepted the food happily, even though they have little interest in adopting this way of eating. Beth spent time cooking with her mom, which they both enjoyed. When her parents visit next time, Beth and her mom are going to pick out and try new recipes together.

In Chapters 11 and 12, we go into more depth about attitudes and behavior change. Read or page through these chapters whenever you feel you need more help in these areas.

Be Empowered

- Pick up a journal or open a computer document to track your lifestyle reset.
- Set aside time to work on your personal wellness vision.
- Create 3-month behavioral goals that will lead you toward your healthiest self.
- Create 1- or 2-week behavioral goals that will lead to success with your 3-month goals.
- Track your progress with the Goal-Tracker on page 269 in Appendix B, electronically or any way that is convenient for you.
- Share your goals and your progress on social media. Use #LifestyleReset and @NutritionJill.

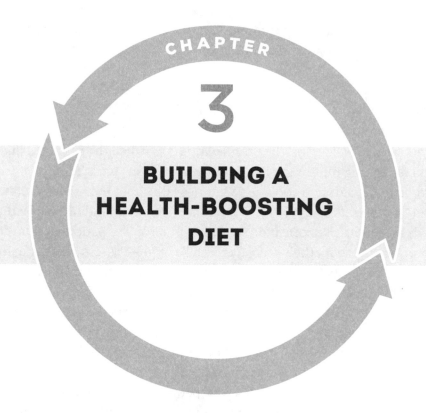

BUILDING A HEALTH-BOOSTING DIET

*A*s mentioned earlier, there are many ways to build a wholesome, disease-fighting diet. There are no hard and fast rules about how many meals and snacks you must eat daily; how many grams of protein, fat, or carbohydrate to include each day; whether you must eat meat or should never eat meat; and so many other diet factors. Many people have strong opinions about what constitutes the ideal diet, but science hasn't yet—and probably never will—identify a single best diet for everyone or a single best diet to prevent diabetes. *Your* best diet is the one that is made up of mostly nutrient-dense, health-boosting foods and is one you enjoy, keeps you energized and satisfied, and is a diet you can stick with.

As you go through this book and implement new strategies, you will find your best diet. Expect your diet to change over time. A complete diet overhaul rarely lasts, but one with gradual (and delicious) changes is more likely to stick.

Foundations of a Health-Boosting Diet

Even without weight loss, healthful eating boosts health. The word "diet" means nothing more than the foods we eat. Everyone then has a diet, and no one needs to be on one. When we talk about being on a diet, we are typically referring to a very restricted food plan and often one that leads to feelings of deprivation. When I ask about my patients' diets, I'm simply asking about their usual food intake. When I assess a diet's healthfulness, I care about what the person usually eats and usually omits.

Often, however, patients are quick to tell me about the foods or ingredients they avoid. They look for foods labeled no added sugars, no artificial sweeteners, low sodium, gluten-free, nonfat, grain-free, and the like. Somewhere in recent decades, avoiding foods and ingredients has become the focus of healthful eating. This scenario is frustrating and sad because so many people avoid what they consider "bad foods" or "bad ingredients," yet they eat so little of the nourishing foods the body optimally runs on and requires to best prevent chronic diseases. For example, fat-free, low-sodium pretzels might be a better snack than cookies, but pretzels don't compare to nuts, fruits, yogurt, hummus, vegetables, and many other nutrient-dense foods. And pretzels will do little to prevent heart disease, type 2 diabetes, or cancer. And just because Americans eat too much added sugar doesn't mean that we have to stop eating *all* added sugars. For all their mouth-puckering tartness, I'd never be able to eat cranberries without some added sweetness. Yogurt too is quite tart. If it takes adding some sugar to enjoy the flavors and health benefits of yogurt and cranberries, I'm all for it. But only when good sense is applied.

In Chapter 4, we'll discuss dietary strategies for weight management, and in Chapter 5, we'll look at various meal-planning techniques. In this chapter, we start with discussing healthful eating in general and food that might be beneficial for diabetes prevention and blood glucose control specifically. That's because I don't want you to fall into the common trap of emphasizing only one health concern. Too often, people focus only on calories for weight, carbs for blood glucose, sodium for blood pressure, or fat for cholesterol. This myopic view of health and diet rarely leads to good outcomes.

The good news is that a healthful diet for diabetes prevention overlaps nicely with dietary strategies for the prevention or treatment of other common health problems such as obesity, stroke, heart disease, colon cancer, and more. These preventive measures are not conflicting with one another as many people believe.

What Does Nutrient-Dense Mean?

Very simply, nutrient-dense foods are foods with lots of nutrients in a small amount or for few calories. Fruits, vegetables, whole grains, beans, nuts, seeds, lean meats, fish, and low-fat and nonfat dairy are nutrient-dense foods. Aside from vitamins, minerals, and fiber, plants also offer phytochemicals or phytonutrients. Scientists have identified thousands of these disease-fighting compounds, and each plant food has its own profile of nutrients and phytonutrients. The only way to get the proper mix is to eat a large variety of plant foods and other nutrient-dense foods in ample quantities. It's not enough to eat a variety of food groups; good nutrition also requires a variety of foods within each food group.

Often, foods marketed as being good for you really aren't. They may be labeled low-fat, grain-free, or sugar-free, but these are not descriptions of nutrient density. These labels simply identify what's not in a food, which may or may not even be important. The bottom line is, look at what's in your food, not just what is missing from your food. Health-boosting foods are nutrient-dense and provide important nutrients and/or phytochemicals that contribute to health and shield you from disease.

Focus on Eating Patterns

In recent years, federal guidelines like the 2015–2020 Dietary Guidelines for Americans, health associations such as the American Diabetes Association, and health care professionals have talked more about dietary patterns or eating patterns and less about individual foods and nutrients. The sum of all the foods and nutrients you eat affects your well-being. The combination and amounts of foods and nutrients you consume interact to work for you or against you. Snacking on wholesome walnuts and almonds, for example, likely has a different effect in the diet of someone who eats greasy fast food and rich desserts daily than it does in the diet of a more health-conscious person.

Of course, dietary patterns are made up of individual foods, so we can't avoid talking about them. We'll cover more about the foods and types of foods that make up wholesome dietary patterns later in this chapter.

Types of Eating Patterns

One study in Finland followed more than 4,000 middle-aged and older men and women for 23 years. Researchers found that the adults who consumed the most fruits and vegetables were the least likely to develop type 2 diabetes. And those who consumed diets rich in butter, potatoes, and whole milk were the most likely to be diagnosed with the disease. This result doesn't prove that butter, potatoes, or whole milk cause diabetes, but it does tell us that differences in dietary patterns matter. After an extensive review, the 2015 Dietary Guidelines Advisory Committee concluded that evidence exists that a *dietary pattern higher in vegetables, fruits, and whole grains and lower in red and processed meats, high-fat dairy products, refined grains, sweets, and sugar-sweetened beverages reduces the risk of developing type 2 diabetes.*

In the following discussion of healthful dietary patterns, you will see many differences. But the similarities are greater than the differences. Wholesome, disease-fighting eating patterns are built around fruits, vegetables, beans, whole grains, nuts, and seeds. That doesn't mean that wholesome diets contain only these foods. Some patterns regularly include fish, dairy, eggs, beef, poultry, and cooking oils. Fortunately, every health-boosting dietary pattern can squeeze in a little of the extra fun stuff, too, like sweets and fried foods.

The typical American diet is full of unhealthful foods and nutrients, including excess calories, saturated fats, added sugars, fatty meats, baked goods, and highly processed grains. The diet tends to be low in fish, fruits, vegetables, whole grains, and beans. This type of eating pattern destroys health and is linked to type 2 diabetes, metabolic syndrome, overweight and obesity, heart disease, and many types of cancer. Whether or not your diet resembles this typical American dietary pattern, chances are good that your diet leaves at least a little room for improvement. And if you become consistent with positive dietary changes, you will experience better health.

As you learn more about dietary patterns or eating patterns to prevent diabetes and other chronic health problems, think about how you will make changes to your own eating pattern. Could you eat less of certain foods and more of others? Can you swap one type of snack for another? Would trimming portions improve your diet? What about cooking at home more often? There are infinite ways to improve your diet. Just keep an open mind as you learn more.

Mediterranean-style diet

People who live in countries surrounding the Mediterranean Sea have traditionally eaten health-promoting diets. Although the typical foods vary from country to country, the basics are the same. The common refrain in this book partly describes a Mediterranean-style diet: choose mostly whole and minimally processed foods and eat lots of vegetables, legumes (like chickpeas, kidney beans, and lentils), fruits, and whole grains. Diets in the Mediterranean region are also rich in nuts, olive oil, and fish. People living there tend to consume wine in moderation and eat bakery items only now and then. Fruit is a common dessert. The diet is not low in fat, but it is fairly low in saturated fats and fairly rich in unsaturated fats. Meals are eaten leisurely, which may help prevent overeating.

Research has linked Mediterranean-style diets to lower risks of developing type 2 diabetes, less incidence of metabolic syndrome, and reduced risks of heart attacks, stroke, and even dementia. A large meta-analysis of more than 100,000 participants from around the world found that individuals whose diets most resembled a Mediterranean-style diet were 23% less likely to develop diabetes. A large study in Spain found that after 4 years, those participants assigned to follow a Mediterranean-style eating pattern were 52% less likely to develop type 2 diabetes than individuals assigned to a low-fat diet. Reduction in risk occurred even without significant weight loss. This information should empower you to focus on healthful food choices whether you lose weight or not. You can learn more about Mediterranean-style diets at Oldways (oldwayspt.org).

DASH diet

DASH stands for Dietary Approaches to Stop Hypertension. This healthful dietary pattern was designed and tested by the National Heart, Lung, and Blood Institute (NHLBI). The DASH diet is rich in fruits, vegetables, low-fat or nonfat dairy, whole grains, poultry, legumes, and nuts. It is low in sodium, added sugars, and saturated fats. It differs from a traditional Mediterranean-style diet by being much lower in fat and richer in dairy products. Although DASH includes more poultry, both diets are rich in plant foods.

The DASH research compared three eating plans: a typical American pattern, the American pattern with additional fruits and vegetables, and the specially devised DASH plan, as described above. Individuals in the extra fruits and vegetables group experienced lowered blood pressure. Those in the DASH group saw their blood pressure levels drop even more. Even when researchers lowered the sodium in the American eating pattern, DASH dropped blood pressure better. Since the development of DASH, researchers have found that it is also linked to less type 2 diabetes, better heart health, and smaller waist sizes. One study found that DASH reduced the risk of developing type 2 diabetes by 20%. Learn more about DASH on the NHLBI website (https://www.nhlbi.nih.gov/health/health-topics/topics/dash).

Vegan diet

A vegan diet omits all animal products. The strictest vegans even avoid honey because bees make it. While a carefully chosen, well-balanced vegan diet is certainly wholesome, a vegan eating pattern is no guarantee of good nutrition. There's no balance in a breakfast of almond milk and cornflakes, a lunch of a peanut butter sandwich, snacks of pretzels and chips, and a dinner of spaghetti and tomato sauce. While this menu is vegan, it is not full of health-boosting fruits, vegetables, whole grains, nuts, and legumes. It is not rich in fiber, phytonutrients, vitamins, potassium, magnesium, unsaturated fats, and more.

Many people at risk for developing type 2 diabetes worry about adopting a vegan diet because of its high carbohydrate content. However, the quantity of carbohydrate is only one part of a diet. The quality of carbohydrate is also important. And a balanced vegan diet rich in disease-fighting foods is no comparison to the pretzel-chip-cornflake diet described above. And it's also no comparison to the typical American diet, which emphasizes unhealthful sources of both fats and carbohydrates. One study found that individuals eating a vegan diet had half the risk of developing type 2 diabetes compared to people eating typical nonvegetarian diets.

Vegetarian diets

There are many variations of a vegetarian diet.

- Ovo vegetarians eat no animal products except eggs.
- Lacto-vegetarians consume dairy products.
- Lacto-ovo vegetarians eat both dairy products and eggs.
- Pescatarians eat fish. They may or may not eat eggs or dairy products.

Regardless of the type of vegetarian diet followed, as long as it is based on wholesome foods, it appears to confer protection against type 2 diabetes and other health problems. Keep in mind that many unhealthful foods such as sugary beverages and cookies are vegetarian. A wholesome diet, however, consists of two parts: ample health-boosting foods and few unhealthful foods. For more information about vegan and vegetarian diets, check out The Vegetarian Resource Group (http://www.vrg.org).

Low-fat or low-carbohydrate diets

Low-fat diets are typically described as containing no more than 30% of total calories as fat. There is no widely accepted description of a low-carb diet. In research studies, some diets described as low-carb contain as little 40 grams carbohydrate per day or as much as 50% of total calories as carbohydrate, which could be much more than 200 grams per day. Having varying definitions of low carb makes comparing research studies difficult. For the most part, however, when it comes to weight loss, low-carb diets win in the short-term. But by the end of a year and beyond, there tends to be little weight loss difference between low-carb diets and other weight loss diets.

A concern about low-fat and low-carb diets is that these plans emphasize what is to be avoided more than what is to be enjoyed. Once I had a patient who came to see me for weight loss and disease prevention. Her diet was very low in fat and also very low in nutrients. She had fully bought into the low-fat dogma of the 1980s and 1990s, even though we were well past those decades. Her diet was full of foods like bread, fat-free pretzels, fat-free ice cream, and fat-free turkey. Even though fruits, vegetables, and legumes are quite low in fat, she wasn't eating much of them. Her diet was terribly unbalanced. Fortunately, she was willing to embrace another way of eating. We reduced the highly processed fat-free foods in her diet and added more whole foods—some with fat and others without. Overall, she consumed more vitamins, minerals, protein, unsaturated fats, and phytonutrients. Her weight dropped, and her energy jumped.

This story speaks to my preference to put more emphasis on the quality of fat rather than the quantity of fat. The original Diabetes Prevention Program recommended a low-fat diet. These days, the American Diabetes Association and other organizations emphasize fat quality over quantity.

The problem with low-carb diets is similar. In recent years, carbohydrates in general and sugar in particular have become common targets for omission. But foods with carbohydrates give us fiber, vitamins, minerals, phytonutrients, plant-based proteins, and more. Carbohydrates are found in vegetables, fruits, whole grains, legumes, milk, yogurt, and even nuts and seeds. Many of these foods contain natural sugars, too. These are precisely the foods linked to good health. I am not pushing a high-carbohydrate diet, but I have strong concerns when people focus on the quantity of carbohydrate over the quality of the food containing carbohydrates. There is good reason to be carb-aware and fat-aware, but there's no reason to be carb- or fat-phobic.

Flexible omnivore diet

An omnivore eats both plants and animals. Most of us are omnivores. My own diet is omnivorous, with mostly wholesome foods and mostly plants. To me, this is the sweet spot for good health, good taste, ease, convenience, and flexibility. In one study, researchers followed more than 200,000 health professionals for more than 2 decades. They learned that even moderately reducing animal foods was associated with less risk for type 2 diabetes. The greatest protection came not from simply reducing meat, but from including mostly healthful plant foods. A plant-rich diet built around mostly health-boosting foods was associated with a 34% reduction in the risk of developing type 2 diabetes. If I were forced to categorize my diet as one of the healthful eating patterns above, I'd label it Mediterranean-style. But because I enjoy a variety of foods and flavors that are not traditional in the Mediterranean region, I say that I have a flexible omnivore diet.

You can learn more about health-boosting eating patterns in the 2015–2020 Dietary Guidelines for Americans (health.gov/dietaryguidelines). Not only should your diet be built around healthful foods, it should be tasty, affordable, and suited to your cultural and religious preferences. Fortunately, there are many ways to do these things. The following graphic shows you two examples. Additionally, you'll find more menu ideas in Chapter 6.

Let Your Plate Be Your Guide

The simple Plate Method is one of the easiest tools to help you build a wholesome meal consistent with any number of healthful eating patterns. Start with a 9-inch plate, and draw an imaginary line down the middle. Fill one-half of the plate with non-starchy vegetables like broccoli, cabbage, tomatoes, carrots, or string beans. Draw another imaginary line across the other half of your plate, so you have two sections equal to one-quarter plate. Put a protein-rich food such as low-fat cottage cheese, black beans, salmon, or lean beef in one section, and a starchy food like corn, peas, quinoa, potato, or brown rice in the last section.

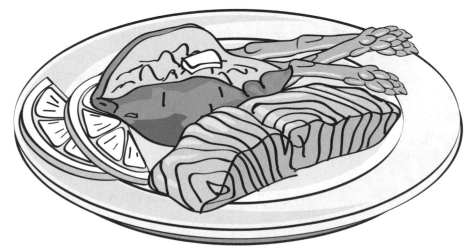

Mediterranean-style plate of salmon, asparagus, and a sweet potato.

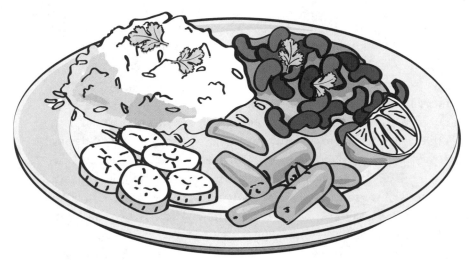

Vegan plate of rice, beans, and a variety of vegetables.

What's the Gut Got to Do with Diabetes?

The gut is home to more than 300 species of bacteria. The number of bacteria in the gut is about 10 times greater than the total number of human cells throughout your body. By some estimates, we are each walking around with at least 3 pounds of gut bacteria. And these bacteria are not just sitting there minding their own business. They are influencing your well-being. Collectively, the microbes residing in the intestines comprise nearly 2 million genes (called the micro-biome). The microbiome is about 100 times greater than the human genome or the number of human genes. When we look at the fact that our bodies have hugely more bacteria genes than human genes, it's not so hard to understand that the bacteria affect health and disease. Indeed, researchers are discovering how intestinal microbes influence obesity, prediabetes and type 2 diabetes, heart disease, and many other illnesses. We have known for a long time that gut microbes synthesize vitamins, break down cancer-causing compounds, release disease-fighting compounds from foods, ferment some types of

(Continued on next page)

fibers and other carbohydrates, and perform many other important roles. But so much more is being studied and learned now.

Some recent studies show that people with obesity have less diverse bacterial species. Individuals with obesity also tend to have more bacteria that are quite good at digesting the remnants of our meals, leaving us to absorb additional calories that would have otherwise been excreted into the stool. So is it possible that having an abundance of this type of bacteria leads to weight gain by making more calories available, or is it possible that being obese leads to more of these bacteria in the intestines? Both are possibilities and may actually occur at the same time. Additionally, the types of predominant bacteria in your intestines may influence inflammation, insulin resistance, and even hormones that help to regulate appetite.

The gut microbiome is far more complicated than this brief description. Scientists continue to untangle the roles bacteria and other microbes play in our health. We also know that the medications we take and the foods we eat greatly affect the types of microbes we harbor in our guts. Studies suggest that a Western-style way of eating (a diet heavy in animal protein, animal fat, refined grains, and added sugars) is associated with a less healthy mix of intestinal bacteria. On the other hand, dietary patterns that include an abundance of whole grains, fruits, vegetables, and legumes are associated with a healthy mix of gut bacteria and health benefits.

Is Your Diet Healthful?

These 19 questions should help you identify some of your dietary strengths and weaknesses. This is not a perfect quiz to determine the healthfulness of your diet. It's simply a way for you to pinpoint an area or two or more to tweak or revamp. Give a second look at each question for which you answer "no" or "sometimes." Then decide if it's an area you want to work on. Some questions may not even apply to you. For example, if you choose a vegan eating pattern, you would not include fish twice weekly. And if you rarely eat between meals, the question about snacks does not concern you. Each of these topics is discussed more fully in later chapters.

1. Do you eat fruits and/or vegetables at most meals, including each breakfast, lunch, and dinner?
   ☐ yes   ☐ no   ☐ sometimes
2. Do you eat at least 1 1/2 cups of vegetables and 1 cup of fruit daily? (Usually more is better.)
   ☐ yes   ☐ no   ☐ sometimes
3. Do you eat the calories and portion sizes that are appropriate for your weight or desired weight?
   ☐ yes   ☐ no   ☐ sometimes
4. Do you eat protein-rich foods like dairy, fish, meat, beans, tofu, or eggs at most meals?
   ☐ yes   ☐ no   ☐ sometimes
5. Do you eat at least three small servings of whole grains daily?
   ☐ yes   ☐ no   ☐ sometimes
6. Do you eat legumes like black beans, lentils, and pinto beans several times per week?
   ☐ yes   ☐ no   ☐ sometimes
7. In a given week, do you eat at least 20 varieties of fruits, vegetables, whole grains, and legumes?
   ☐ yes   ☐ no   ☐ sometimes
8. Do you eat fatty fish like salmon, tuna, lake trout, and herring a couple of times each week?
   ☐ yes   ☐ no   ☐ sometimes
9. When you snack, do you typically choose nutrient-dense foods like nuts, fruits, yogurt, and vegetables?
   ☐ yes   ☐ no   ☐ sometimes
10. Do you limit animal fats and solid fats like fatty cuts of meat, bacon grease, butter, and coconut oil?
    ☐ yes   ☐ no   ☐ sometimes

11. Do you recognize and listen to your body's hunger and fullness cues?

☐ yes　　☐ no　　☐ sometimes

12. When cooking, do you use liquid oils like canola oil more than solid spreads and semi-solid oils like butter, stick margarine, and coconut oil?

☐ yes　　☐ no　　☐ sometimes

13. Do you favor flavorful herbs and spices over salt in your food?

☐ yes　　☐ no　　☐ sometimes

14. Do you avoid sugary drinks like regular sodas and sweet teas?

☐ yes　　☐ no　　☐ sometimes

15. Do you drink alcohol in moderation (defined as no more than 1 drink daily for women and no more than 2 drinks daily for men) if you drink alcohol at all?

☐ yes　　☐ no　　☐ sometimes

16. Do you limit highly processed foods like most chips, snack bars, and white bread?

☐ yes　　☐ no　　☐ sometimes

17. When you eat sweets, fried foods, and other "treat foods," do you limit your portion?

☐ yes　　☐ no　　☐ sometimes

18. When shopping for groceries, do you read food labels to determine the healthfulness of your foods?

☐ yes　　☐ no　　☐ sometimes

19. Do you eat with attention to your food, so you experience pleasure from your meal?

☐ yes　　☐ no　　☐ sometimes

Specific Foods for Diabetes Prevention

Compared to eating a typical American diet, any of the health-boosting eating patterns above will likely bring about a healthier you. In general, keep this in mind: various phytonutrients likely act

A Diet for Longevity

In his book *The Blue Zones*, National Geographic explorer Dan Buettner tells of his travels around the globe to identify the diets, habits, and attitudes of the world's longest-living populations. Buettner and teams of scientists visited five communities in which people celebrated their 100th birthdays at rates 10 times greater than in the U.S. Although the specific foods available and eaten varied based on location, the researchers learned that the diets of each of these healthy populations had a plant slant. While they may eat meat, the focus is on fruits, vegetables, and beans.

in the intestines to slow down glucose absorption and act in other areas of the body to affect glucose metabolism and increase insulin sensitivity. There are probably both short- and long-term actions, so it's smart to eat plant foods with most meals and snacks. Whether or not the above diets will help you lose weight will depend on your total calorie intake and expenditure. Chapter 4 goes into more detail on weight loss.

Some specific foods and other dietary factors are also linked to less risk of type 2 diabetes and better blood glucose control. But even in well-designed research studies, it's hard to tease out the reasons some foods appear to be beneficial and the people most likely to benefit. A food may reduce the risk of disease because when people eat it, they eat less of another food. For instance, when people snack on nuts, they are less likely to snack on candy bars, and when people eat more beans for supper, they may eat less pizza. Plus, the phytonutrients in fruits, vegetables, nuts, and other plants interact with other nutrients and our gut bacteria. So people with different bacteria populations may respond differently to the same foods. Here are some foods to include in your diabetes prevention dietary pattern.

Oats

Oats are a whole grain and contain the soluble fiber β-glucan. β-Glucan improves insulin action and lowers blood glucose levels and also sweeps cholesterol from your digestive tract before it reaches your bloodstream. Hence, oats may help lower your risks for both heart disease and type 2 diabetes.

Barley

Barley also contains cholesterol-lowering, insulin-sensitizing β-glucan.

Legumes and Pulses (Beans, Peas, Lentils)

You know they're good for the heart, but beans are also good for diabetes and diabetes prevention. Both legumes and pulses are studied for their health effects. Because you'll see both words in the news and because they tend to be confusing, I'll define them here. Legumes are the plants in which fruit is enclosed in a pod. Common legumes are soybeans, black beans, chickpeas, kidney beans, and lentils. Pulses are part of the legume family, but they refer only to the dried seed. Pulses include split peas, chickpeas, lentils, and dried beans like kidney beans, black beans, and pinto beans. Soybeans, including tofu and edamame, are legumes, but they are not also pulses. Don't let the choice of word in a news report confuse you. Just know that all of these plant-rich proteins are good for you and are worth seeking out. Studies show that diets rich in legumes have beneficial effects on both short- and long-term fasting blood glucose levels. Not only are they full of plant protein, they contain potassium, magnesium, B vitamins, and dietary fiber, including a special type called "resistant starch." As the name suggests, resistant starches resist digestion in the small intestine. Instead, they travel to the colon where they feed our gut bacteria. In the process, the beneficial bacteria produce short-chain fatty acids that seem to protect the colon cells, make the gut environment more suitable for the friendly bacteria and less suitable for their harmful cousins, and even improve the way our bodies respond to insulin.

Other Sources of Resistant Starches

Legumes are not the only foods with this source of beneficial non-digested carbohydrate. Under-ripe or green bananas contain it. So do uncooked oats (think muesli over cottage cheese or yogurt), brown rice, and potatoes and pasta that have been cooked and cooled (a great reason to enjoy a small serving of potato salad or pasta salad). The U.S. Food and Drug Administration (FDA) recently approved a qualified health claim regarding a specific resistant starch that manufacturers may now put on food labels. You might see labels with the following claim: "High-amylose maize resistant starch may reduce the risk of type 2 diabetes, although FDA has concluded that there is limited scientific evidence for this claim." Although wordy and somewhat confusing, this statement means that there's some pretty good evidence that high-amylose maize resistant starch helps prevent type 2 diabetes, but the evidence is not 100% solid. Food manufacturers may add high-amylose maize resistant starch (or other types of resistant starch) to products such as pasta, pretzels, snack bars, and breads.

Nuts

Some studies show that when people with type 2 diabetes consume nuts, their blood glucose levels improve, as do measures of their heart health. Although not seen in all research, many studies show that eating nuts also helps prevent type 2 diabetes. Very likely, the benefit depends on the total diet. Just like every fruit and every vegetable has a unique profile of nutrients and phytonutrients, each nut is also unique. In general, nuts provide unsaturated fats, vegetable protein, fiber, folate, magnesium, and a host of other vitamins and minerals. Don't fall for the trap that you should eat only one type of nut. Enjoy them all. Almonds give us a good dose of vitamin E. Pistachios have lots of blood pressure–friendly potassium and lutein, which is an antioxidant. Walnuts are the ones with omega-3 fatty acids, and peanuts tend to be easier on the budget than other nuts, even though they are packed with nutrition, too. Keep portions in mind, however, because nuts are calorie dense. Good news on the calorie topic, though: Research has shown that both walnuts and almonds may actually give us fewer calories than the packages say. That's probably because we don't fully digest the nuts, leaving some of those calories to be excreted in the feces. On average, we absorb 21% fewer calories from walnuts and 17–25% fewer calories from almonds. The calories from almond butter are fully absorbed. It's possible that other nuts behave similarly in our digestive tracts, but we don't have the research to know for sure.

Whole Grains

Because there are so many types of whole grains and so many ways to eat them, researching them as a group is confusing. However, according to the 2015 Dietary Guidelines Advisory Committee, healthful patterns that include whole grains appear to be associated with less type 2 diabetes. Here are some examples of whole grains:

- Whole wheat
- Wheat berries
- Farro
- Freekeh
- Sorghum
- Amaranth
- Whole rye
- Oats, oatmeal, rolled oats
- Whole-grain corn
- Whole-grain barley

- Wild rice
- Brown rice
- Millet
- Popcorn
- Quinoa

Unsaturated Fats

We hear a lot about avoiding trans fats and saturated fats for the sake of our hearts. Research shows that when we replace these unhealthful fatty acids with either unsaturated fats or wholesome sources of carbohydrates, our risk for heart disease drops. Switching to the more healthful monounsaturated and polyunsaturated fats appears to boost insulin sensitivity, too. A Mediterranean-style diet is typically rich in monounsaturated fatty acids and low in saturated fats. A few sources of unsaturated fats include the following:

- Olive, canola, and peanut oils
- Tree nuts and peanuts, nut butters
- Avocados
- Olives

We'll cover more about dietary fats in Chapters 4 and 6.

Yogurt

Although studies are mixed, many suggest that dairy foods have a protective effect against type 2 diabetes. Perhaps the strongest link is the association between yogurt and less risk of diabetes. One large population study found that an increase of one serving of yogurt per day was associated with an 18% lower risk of developing type 2 diabetes. It's unclear how yogurt could influence health this way, but it may be related to its probiotics or unique nutritional profile. Some studies also link yogurt to lower obesity risk.

Berries

A Finnish study found that middle-aged and older men who consumed the most berries had a whopping 35% lower risk of developing type 2 diabetes. Enjoy a variety. Choose strawberries, blueberries, raspberries, and others.

Fruits

In general, eating fruits is associated with less chronic disease, not more. Yet many people fear fruit because of its carbohydrate content. Specifically, most of the carbohydrate in fruit is sugar, so it's not surprising why many people worry. While it is true that carbohydrate raises blood glucose levels more than other nutrients, it is not true that fruit raises blood glucose more than other carb-containing foods. It's important to recognize that foods are much more than their macronutrient (carbohydrate, protein, and fat) content. Avoiding carbohydrate because it raises blood glucose is like throwing the baby out with the bathwater. Fruits, along with other plant foods, contain so many disease-fighting, insulin-sensitizing compounds that it's a bad idea to forgo them.

Herbs and Spices

These flavor boosters provide us with the same types of disease-fighting phytonutrients that are in fruits and vegetables. Add taste with both fresh and dried seasonings. Cinnamon in particular has been studied for its potential effects on blood glucose levels. Add some to oatmeal, cottage cheese, yogurt, and even coffee.

Vinegar

Research suggests that vinegar consumed with a high-carbohydrate meal improves both blood glucose and insulin levels. Sprinkle some on your salad, roasted vegetables, and other foods.

Coffee

Several studies link drinking coffee (decaffeinated or regular) to less risk of developing type 2 diabetes. But it's important to consider how you prepare and drink your coffee. Unfiltered coffee, such as coffee made with a French press, contains cafestol and kahweol, compounds that raise LDL (bad) cholesterol levels. Filtering your coffee with a paper filter removes these harmful compounds. Keep your coffee low-calorie and healthful by drinking it plain or with a splash of milk. A heavy hand with syrups, sugars, and cream will turn your coffee into quite a nutritional goof.

Tea

Drinking tea may also shield you from type 2 diabetes. One analysis suggests that the more tea an individual drinks, the greater the benefit, with as little as 1 cup per day dropping the risk of developing the disease by 3%. Again, pay attention to what you put into your tea to avoid excess calories, added sugars, and saturated fats.

Alcohol

Consuming small amounts of alcohol is also linked to less type 2 diabetes. But alcohol in excess is linked to more, as well as many other problems. That's why the American Diabetes Association and other organizations do not recommend drinking for the prevention of disease. If you do drink, you don't need much. The benefits of drinking alcohol appear to occur with as little as one-half standard drink daily. Consuming alcohol in moderation is also associated with reduced risk of dying from heart disease. Alcohol might protect the heart by increasing HDL (good) cholesterol. Additionally, the phytonutrients and other antioxidant compounds in red wine may further benefit the heart by protecting the blood vessels from oxidative damage. Remember that moderate drinking is defined as no more than one drink daily for women and no more than two drinks daily for men. And the size of those drinks matters. What we pour ourselves or receive in bars and restaurants is often much more than a single standard drink.

What Counts as One Drink?	
Alcoholic Beverage	**Amount**
Beer	12 fluid ounces
	1 bottle or can
Liquor such as bourbon and vodka	1.5 fluid ounces of 80-proof liquor
	1 fluid ounce of 100-proof liquor
Wine	5 fluid ounces

Bottom Line

Once again, the bottom line is that a dietary pattern or an eating pattern to prevent type 2 diabetes is a general health-boosting diet. Build your diet around a variety of foods and food groups with an emphasis on whole plant foods.

Be Empowered

- Commit to a diet rich in whole foods and relatively low in refined and highly processed foods. It's okay to make gradual changes.
- Assess your diet with the quiz on page 54. Then pick two to five small dietary changes to work on. Create SMART goals around your selected dietary changes.
- Using the list of foods that are associated with less risk of diabetes, create your weekly grocery list. See Chapter 6 for smart shopping tips.

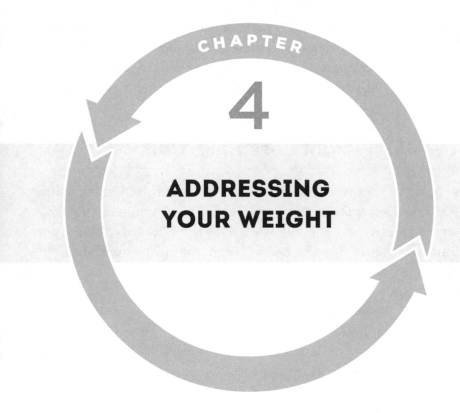

CHAPTER

4

ADDRESSING YOUR WEIGHT

*U*sually (although not always), prediabetes is associated with extra body fat. If you are overweight, losing even a few pounds can improve your health. As discussed in Chapter 1, the results of the Diabetes Prevention Program and other research studies tell us that weight loss can help prevent or delay the onset of type 2 diabetes.

If your goal is better health, you do not need to lose huge amounts of weight. Dropping a few pounds can have profound benefit. In a fascinating study among people at high risk for developing type 2 diabetes, losing only 5% of body weight (10 pounds for someone starting at 200 pounds) improved insulin sensitivity in the fat, muscle, and liver cells. This small weight loss also improved the function of the pancreas β-cells (the cells that produce insulin) and reduced the amount of fat in the liver. As weight loss continued first to 11% and then to 16% of starting weight, the participants experienced greater improvements. Their muscle cells became even more sensitive to insulin, they lost more fat from their livers, and the function of their β-cells improved even more. So even if you don't see the positive effects of weight loss, they are likely occurring under the surface.

How Will Weight Loss Help You?

Preventing diabetes must be near the top of your list, but it's unlikely to be your only reason to lose weight. The benefits are really too many to identify, but the following is a pretty good list. Spend a few minutes with it to find the reasons that are most important to you. You can create your list in your journal or a notebook or simply put a checkmark next to the benefits that matter most. Having a personalized list will help you with motivation, which commonly goes up and down and often without obvious reason. You will see that I've included benefits unrelated to your physical health. That's because there are many powerful reasons to lose weight that are more emotional in nature.

- Lower insulin resistance, improve β-cell function, and reduce my risk for type 2 diabetes
- Improve my cholesterol and triglyceride levels
- Lower my blood pressure
- Reduce systemic inflammation, which is linked to chronic diseases like type 2 diabetes and heart disease
- Lower my risk for some types of cancer
- Improve sleep apnea
- Possibly reduce or discontinue some medications or prevent the addition of others
- Have less urinary incontinence
- Suffer less knee or back pain
- Increase fertility
- Feel more energetic

- Feel more confident
- Enjoy physical activity
- Enjoy shopping for clothing
- Be more comfortable crossing legs, sitting on the floor, etc.
- Improve sleep
- Be a good role model
- Other: _____
- Other: _____
- Other: _____

When You're DONE Trying to Lose Weight

I've known many people who have spent a lifetime trying to lose weight. They may have followed many strict diet plans to lose weight, only to gain it back when they end the diet. They repeat this cycle until they can no longer tolerate another weight loss plan. If your experience is similar and you've given up trying to lose weight, you can still benefit from living healthfully. Your weight is not everything when it comes to good health. While it is certainly important, there are many important lifestyle habits for you to focus your efforts and energy on. You'll find them in each of the chapters of this book. Committing to healthful living and avoiding further weight gain are important and admirable goals. You may find that your motivation for weight loss inches upward as time goes on anyway. And if not, you're still ahead by maintaining your current weight, being active, eating healthfully, tending to stress, and otherwise living healthfully.

Assessing Weight

Although we think of fat tissue as being inert blobs just sitting on our waist and hips, fat is actually very busy, metabolically speaking. Fat cells secrete hormones and other chemicals that create chronic low levels of inflammation. The amount of excess body fat you have is associated with your risk for prediabetes, type 2 diabetes, heart disease, gallstones, gastroesophageal reflux disorder, and some types of cancer.

There are several sophisticated ways to learn how much body fat you have, including magnetic resonance imaging (MRI) and dual-energy X-ray absorptiometry. These procedures are not practical for the average person and are typically reserved for research studies. When done properly, however, skinfold thickness measurements are very revealing. They are especially helpful as a tool to track your progress with a fitness or weight loss routine. If you belong to a gym or health club, there may be a trained fitness instructor capable of estimating your body fatness with skinfold measurements.

Health care professionals and researchers, however, typically assess weight with two quick measurements: body mass index (or BMI) and waist circumference.

Body Mass Index (BMI)

Body mass index is derived from a simple calculation based on your height and weight. It alone cannot identify your health risk or your level of body fatness. But it's a pretty good tool to estimate your risk for weight-related health problems, including type 2 diabetes. In general, the higher your BMI, the greater your risk. BMI tends to overestimate body fatness in athletes and others who are very muscular, and it underestimates levels of body fat in individuals who have little muscle.

To quickly find your BMI, visit the website of the Centers for Disease Control and Prevention (CDC) or the National Heart, Lung, and Blood Institute (NHLBI). Both sites have BMI calculators that require nothing more than knowing your height and weight. You can also calculate your own with the following formula:

$$BMI = \text{Weight in pounds}/\text{height in inches}^2 \times 703.$$

Example: Bob weighs 200 pounds and is 5'10" tall (70 inches tall). Bob's BMI = $200/70^2 \times 703 = 28.7 \text{ kg/m}^2$. According to the chart below, Bob is classified as overweight.

How To Interpret Your BMI

The following chart is for adults only. For help in understanding your child's BMI, talk to a health care professional.

BMI (kg/m²)	Weight Status
<18.5	Underweight
18.5–24.9	Normal or Healthy Weight
25.0–29.9	Overweight
≥30.0	Obese

It is worth noting that research suggests that Asian Americans have increased health risks beginning at a lower BMI. For this reason, some organizations classify a healthy weight for Asian Americans at a BMI of 18.5–22.9 kg/m², an overweight BMI between 23 and 26.9 kg/m², and an obese BMI at ≥27 kg/m².

Waist Circumference

A second measure to categorize obesity and risk is your waist size. Excess body fat can land anywhere in the body, but research suggests that the fat around our midsections is especially harmful. The terms "belly fat" and "visceral fat" mean the same thing. Fat that accumulates around the internal organs can actually infiltrate these organs, causing fatty liver and excess fat in the pancreas, heart, and other organs not suited to fat storage.

How to measure your waist circumference

As a woman, I want to put my hands on the smallest part of my midsection and call that my waist. But this is not the proper location for an accurate assessment. My tape measure needs to be a bit lower. Follow these steps.

1. While standing, place a tape measure around your midsection directly above the tip of your hipbones.
2. Be sure that your tape measure is horizontal.
3. Breathe out normally and measure. Be careful that the tape measure is snug against your skin, but is not compressing your skin.

The NHLBI categorizes high risk as a waist measurement >40 inches for men and >35 inches for women. Interestingly, however, the American Institute for Cancer Research (AICR) finds that smaller waist sizes confer increased risk for many types of cancer. To lower the risk of a variety of cancers, the AICR recommends that men have waist sizes no larger than 37 inches and that women aim for waists of no more than 31.5 inches. And some ethnic populations may have an increased risk at even lower waist measurements. The Joslin Diabetes Center identifies target waistline goals for Asian American women at no more than 31.5 inches and no more than 35.5 inches for Asian American men.

Pick a Weight Loss Goal

Before vowing to reach your dream weight, consider all that you have just read. Any weight loss is better than none. Losing even as little as 5% of your starting weight has profound health benefits, as you saw in the study mentioned above. Plus, the amount of weight you keep off long term is much more important than the amount of weight you lose in the short term. I often tell my patients that I don't care how much weight they lose; I care how much weight they keep off.

I encourage you to pick a modest weight loss goal. The goal for the DPP was to lose 7% of starting weight, but you should start with whatever reasonable goal you feel is right for you. Once you reach it, you can always pick a second goal, and then a third goal, and so on. Depending on many factors, including your starting weight and physical activity level, you will likely be able to drop 5–10% of your weight in 3–6 months. You can keep track of your weight on the chart on page 272 in Appendix B, in your journal, or on a smartphone app.

Your Weight (pounds)	5–10% (pounds)	New Goal Weight (pounds)
120	6–12	108–114
140	7–14	126–133
160	8–16	144–152
180	9–18	162–171
200	10–20	180–190
220	11–22	198–209
240	12–24	216–228
260	13–26	234–247
280	14–28	252–266
300	15–30	270–285
320	16–32	288–304
340	17–34	306–323
360	18–36	324–342
380	19–38	342–361
400	20–40	360–380
420	21–42	378–399

Weight Loss Basics

Just as I've said that there are many ways to a healthy plate, there are many ways to achieve weight loss. This chapter will review the basics. For individualized help, I recommend working with a registered dietitian nutritionist (RD or RDN). You can find one in your local area by visiting the website of the Academy of Nutrition and

Dietetics (eatright.org) and entering your zip code after clicking on the "Find an Expert" tab.

Understanding Fats, Carbohydrates, Protein, and Calories

Fats, carbohydrates, and protein are macronutrients. Other than alcohol, these are the only nutrients that provide calories. Gram for gram, fat provides more than twice the calories of either protein or carbohydrate. There's been a lot of debate over the years about which of these macronutrients should be restricted or emphasized in the diet to achieve the greatest weight loss. Some people have very strong opinions about low-fat or low-carb diets and can likely find good research to support their position. But there is research to support a variety of opinions. It's important to look at the preponderance of the evidence before picking a side to stand firm.

When I look at the evidence as a whole, I see that a lot of diet types work. So much of it has to do with your preference. Generally, low-carb diets lead to more weight loss in the short term. But when studies last a year or longer, low-carb plans tend to produce no more and no less weight loss than other types of diets. The most important factor appears to be how adherent the dieter is to the plan. My preference is not to emphasize protein, fat, or carbohydrate. When we do so, I think we get lost in a bunch of gobbledygook that really makes no difference in the long run. I prefer instead to look at the food quality. That makes a difference in the short term and the long term. I emphasize fruits, vegetables, legumes, and whole grains over pretzels, white bread, soda, cookies, and toaster pastries—although all are rich in carbohydrates. When it comes to fats, I encourage foods rich in unsaturated fats like nuts, liquid oils, fatty fish, and avocado over butter, bacon grease, fatty meats, and baked goods, which are all sources of less healthful saturated fats. And when it comes to protein sources, I emphasize those that are lean, such as skinless poultry and low-fat dairy; contain heart-healthy fats, such as salmon and tuna;

The Macronutrients

Macronutrient	Notes
Carbohydrate **Fiber:** A type of carbohydrate with many physiological benefits, including for colon health, cholesterol metabolism, and glucose metabolism. **Sugar:** Small carbohydrate molecules, found naturally in fruit, vegetables, and milk. Excessive *added* sugars are a problem for health. **Starch:** Larger carbohydrate molecules found in grains, legumes, and some vegetables.	Provides 4 calories per gram (except for fiber and sugar alcohols). Only carbohydrate-containing foods contain dietary fiber. Carbohydrates have a greater effect on blood glucose levels after a meal compared to fats and protein.
Fat **Polyunsaturated fat:** A type of unsaturated fat that when consumed in place of saturated and trans fats provides health benefits. It is common in nuts, salad dressings, and fatty fish. **Monounsaturated fat:** A second type of unsaturated fat that when consumed in place of saturated and trans fats confers health benefits. It is common in olive and canola oils, olives, and avocados. **Saturated fat:** Tends to raise LDL (bad) cholesterol levels and may increase insulin resistance. Saturated fat is found in animal fats, dairy fat, and solid and semi-solid fats like coconut oil and other tropical oils.	Provides 9 calories per gram. Consuming fat with your meals helps you absorb fat-soluble vitamins and phytonutrients. Experts recommend consuming only 5–10% of total calories from saturated fats, which could be as little as 8 grams daily on a 1,400-calorie diet and as much as 22 grams daily on a 2,000-calorie diet.

(Continued on next page)

Macronutrient	Notes
Trans fat: A type of unhealthful fat that is linked to heart disease and type 2 diabetes. It's created when food manufacturers partially hydrogenate oils to make packaged foods more shelf-stable. Trans fats may also be in fried foods.	Try not to eat factory-produced trans fats, and avoid anything with *partially* hydrogenated oils.
Protein Protein is made up of essential and nonessential amino acids. The greatest sources of protein are all types of meat, milk, yogurt, cheese, and legumes. Vegetables, nuts, and grains also provide some protein.	Provides 4 calories per gram. Of the three macronutrients, protein tends to help control appetite best. Recent research tells us that spreading protein out over the day helps with body composition. Instead of eating small amounts at breakfast and lunch and piling on the protein at dinner, eat more moderate portions at each of your three meals to better stimulate muscle synthesis.

and are plant-based, such as lentils, tofu, and kidney beans. The truth is, most foods are sources of more than one of these macronutrients. For example, black beans provide both carbohydrates and protein. And salmon is a source of both protein and fat. Even olive and peanut oils, rich in unsaturated fats, contain some saturated fats, too. Without focusing on one macronutrient over another, it's possible (and easier) to choose nutrient-dense, disease-fighting foods.

Calories Do Count

Without burning more calories than you consume, you cannot lose weight. There is a big difference in healthfulness between weight loss diets that consist primarily of lollipops and gumdrops and those consisting of a variety of whole foods. But even the unhealthful diet will result in weight loss if the calories are low enough. Indeed, we have seen the results of such a diet in the media when a university professor put himself on a calorie-restricted diet that contained little more than snack cakes, chips, cookies, and sugary cereals. Because he kept his calorie intake to less than 1,800 per day, he lost a significant amount of weight in just 2 months. The media also reported on a high school teacher who subsisted on a variety of foods from McDonald's for 6 months and lost more than 50 pounds. These stories demonstrate that calories do indeed count.

This does not mean, however, that you need to count calories to make them count for you. You can trim calories from your diet and burn a few more during physical activity without ever having to count them. Most of my own patients and clients find that it's helpful to get an idea of where their calories come from, so they may keep a calorie tally for a few days or longer. Others just need a ballpark idea.

While there are sophisticated formulas to estimate your calorie needs, you probably don't need to break out your calculator. I favor the approach researchers took in the large federally funded Look AHEAD (Action for Health in Diabetes) trial, a weight loss study among people with type 2 diabetes. They didn't use formulas or any fancy algorithm. They simply assigned a range of 1,200–1,500 calories daily to individuals weighing less than 250 pounds and a range of 1,500–1,800 calories daily to individuals who started the program weighing more than 250 pounds. If you are very active, you likely need more calories than if you are sedentary or only moderately active, so keep that in mind. For something more individualized, check out the Adults Energy Needs Calculator on the website of Baylor College of Medicine (https://www.bcm.edu/cnrc-apps/caloriesneed.cfm). You can also work with a registered dietitian nutritionist.

Metabolic Rate

Your metabolic rate is the rate at which your body uses calories. You will lose weight when you consume fewer calories than your body uses. Weight loss really is a numbers game. Unfortunately, the numbers game is complicated, so weight loss is rarely in a straight line. There is much about the body that we don't understand. We don't know why some people can cut calories and lose more weight than another person who appears to trim calories similarly. We don't fully understand why sometimes lost weight so readily comes back. And we don't know why some people boost exercise, consume fewer calories, and appear resistant to weight loss. There are hormonal changes, metabolic adaptations, and unknown factors that occur with weight loss or food restriction that make it harder for some people to lose weight and maintain that weight loss.

But we do understand what metabolic rate is, and there are three components to it:

1. *Basal metabolic rate.* This is the largest portion of your metabolic rate, accounting for about two-thirds of your daily calorie expenditure. These are the calories used to keep you alive and tend to basic bodily functions like breathing, maintaining body temperature, circulating blood, and repairing cells. Your weight and body composition drive your basal metabolic rate. The bigger you are, the greater your basal metabolic rate. When you lose weight, your basal metabolic rate drops.

2. *Food processing.* It takes calories to digest, absorb, and assimilate nutrients from food. This smallest component of your metabolic rate is referred to as the thermic effect of food (TEF). Contrary to some information, you do not burn more calories through the TEF by eating more often. The TEF is related to what you eat, not how many times you eat. If, for example, you consume 1,500 calories in three meals per day or eat that same food over six meals per day, your 24-hour metabolic rate will not differ.

3. *Physical activity.* You have the most control here. The more active you are, the more calories you burn. Activity includes both exercise for the purpose of exercise and physical activities of daily living—things like folding laundry, walking to answer the phone, fidgeting, etc.

Do Metabolism Boosters Work?

You've probably seen a long list of foods or tricks that supposedly rev your metabolic motor. Some are downright false. Others cause such a tiny spike in metabolic rate that they become more of a distraction to establishing healthful habits than a benefit to a weight loss plan. In short-term studies, both caffeine and spicy peppers boost metabolic rate slightly, but neither one has demonstrated long-term weight loss. When you drink very cold water, the body uses about an extra 12 calories to warm it up. That's hardly enough to force yourself to drink icy water. Eating extra protein, sipping green tea, and taking supplements all make the list of diet tricks. Unfortunately, weight loss supplements are often dangerous, so I do not recommend them ever. The others are typically minimally helpful at best. My biggest gripe with these "metabolism-boosting tricks" is that they steer energy, focus, and effort to all the wrong places. Skip these time-wasters. You are much better off putting effort and time into meal planning, physical activity, visiting a farmer's market, and eating mindfully.

Be Calorie Aware

If you choose to count calories for a few days or longer, you'll need to read food labels, use measuring utensils, have a calorie database at your fingertips, and do a bit of math. There are many suitable calorie databases available, including the app LoseIt. When I'm looking for specific restaurant information, I use my web browser to search for the name of the restaurant and the word nutrition. For example, you'll find what you want to know about your food at Panera Bread by searching for "Panera Bread nutrition." Do the same for any chain restaurant.

Even if you choose not to track and record your calorie intake, it's still important to be aware of calories. Say your goal is to eat about 1,500–1,800 calories per day. It's smart to identify foods in your diet that are high in calories and low in calories. Make an effort to eat more that are low and fewer that are high. When you read a food label or look up a food in your database, ask yourself how does it fit into a healthful 1,500- to 1,800-calorie eating plan. That candy bar may not be delicious and satisfying enough for 240 calories once you learn that you can eat 3 chocolate kisses and a cup of light yogurt for fewer calories—and more nutrition.

Use Food Labels for Calorie Information

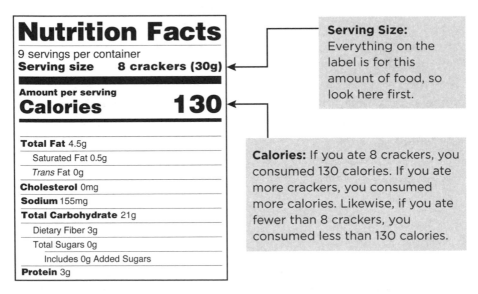

Nutrition Facts

9 servings per container
Serving size   8 crackers (30g)

Amount per serving
Calories   130

Total Fat 4.5g
    Saturated Fat 0.5g
    Trans Fat 0g
Cholesterol 0mg
Sodium 155mg
Total Carbohydrate 21g
    Dietary Fiber 3g
    Total Sugars 0g
        Includes 0g Added Sugars
Protein 3g

Serving Size: Everything on the label is for this amount of food, so look here first.

Calories: If you ate 8 crackers, you consumed 130 calories. If you ate more crackers, you consumed more calories. Likewise, if you ate fewer than 8 crackers, you consumed less than 130 calories.

Don't confuse the serving size on a food label as your portion size. You may serve yourself more or less food than the amount shown on the label as a single serving. The example above is fairly simple because you can count the exact number of crackers you eat. Sixteen crackers give you 260 calories. Eating only 4 crackers means you consume only 65 calories. And my calculator tells me that 10 crackers serve up about 163 calories. Consider how the total amount of calories in your portion of food fits into your total calorie allotment.

It's not so easy to determine the portion size of most foods. You'll need measuring cups for juice, soup, rice, and more. And you'll need measuring spoons for cooking oils, salad dressings, and other condiments. A food scale may also be helpful.

Be Portion Savvy

I always say that nearly any food can fit into a healthful eating plan if the portion is small enough. I also warn my patients that even the most healthful foods can't be eaten in unlimited quantities. Brown rice, nuts, and salmon are all wholesome, health-boosting foods, but if you ate them with abandon, you'd likely pack on some weight. Try these 11 portion control strategies.

- *Use small dishes.* Your smaller portions won't look so tiny on a small plate or bowl. Serve lunch and dinner on 9-inch plates. Ladle hearty soups into cups that hold about 1 cup and brothy soups into bowls that hold slightly more. Look for 1/2-cup dishes for ice cream and other desserts.
- *Purchase portion-control dishes.* Portion-control dishes are easy to find in department stores, online, and in discount stores. With their innovative designs, they guide you to serve up the perfect portion. A few to look for include Fit & Fresh, Livliga, Precise Portions, and Slimware.
- *Weigh and measure everything you eat for 5–7 days.* Weighing and measuring your portion sizes will give you a sense of the amount of food you eat. Then each month, periodically weigh and measure everything again for a day or two to ensure that a 1/3-cup serving hasn't expanded to 1/2 cup and a 1-cup serving didn't grow to 1 1/2 cups. Recently, a patient reported sticking to her

calorie goal, but admitted to not measuring her foods. When her weight didn't budge, she agreed to measure everything for 1 week. That's when her weight came down. She was eating more than she realized.

- *Treat yourself to foods in single-serving portions.* Skip the half-gallon containers of ice cream in favor of ice cream bars or sandwiches. Better yet, treat yourself now and then to a small cone or cup at a local ice cream parlor.
- *Pre-portion tempting foods.* Place crackers, chips, nuts, cookies, and other tempting foods into small containers or baggies to make selecting the proper portion completely effortless.
- *Ask for help.* I nearly always have someone else serve me dessert, so I'm not tempted to take a large portion. I also frequently ask my daughter to frost birthday cakes to help keep me off chocolate frosting until it's time to cut the cake.
- *Eat only from a dish.* No reaching into a bag or a box and eating some unknown amount. Put a measured amount of food into a bowl, onto a plate, or even onto a napkin.
- *Serve dinner from the kitchen counter.* By serving meats and starches from the counter instead of the table, you deter second helpings. On the other hand, leave fruits and vegetables in easy-to-reach places to encourage eating more of these foods.
- *Fill up on low-calorie foods.* With more vegetables satisfying your appetite, you'll have less need to eat large portions of higher-calorie foods.
  - Eat fruits and vegetables at every meal and snack.
  - Enjoy a glass of tomato or vegetable juice before a meal.
  - Start your meal with a broth-based soup, a low-calorie vegetable salad, or a few steamed shrimp.
- *Slow down.* Sip water; enjoy the conversation; focus on the flavors, textures, and aromas of your food; put your fork down

between bites; or use small utensils like an espresso spoon to eat ice cream, yogurt, and puddings.

- *Try a low-calorie, portion-controlled meal.* Research shows that meal replacements and portion-controlled meals can help with weight loss. Eating them now and then can help you relearn appropriate portions. Add a salad, some vegetables, or both to give you more nutrition and help you feel full longer. Here are a few guidelines (not hard and fast rules) to help you pick a prepared meal.
  - No more than 400 calories, 3 grams saturated fat, and 600 mg sodium
  - No trans fats at all
  - At least 3 grams fiber, but preferably 5 or more
  - At least 14 grams protein, but 25 is better

Know Your Hunger

A lot of things trigger us to eat and to overeat. Maybe you're in the habit of having a snack when your kids come home from school. Watching TV commercials about food sends some people to the kitchen. And simply seeing candy in a candy dish prompts others to eat. Or happy, sad, or uncomfortable feelings provoke eating. Ideally, we eat to satisfy our hunger or to prevent being over-hungry later. For example, if dinner will be late, I often eat a snack around 5:00 P.M. when I break from my work. A piece of fruit, some reduced-fat cheese, or leftover vegetables give me a nutritional boost and keep me from being ravenous later.

To help you recognize your hunger and fullness signals and to help you learn the appropriate amount of food to eat, experiment with the Hunger Ruler below. Before, during, and after your meals, record the number that corresponds to your hunger. It's good to start your meal when you are a bit hungry (level 3 or 4) and stop eating when you are no longer hungry and just full enough (level 6).

Hunger Ruler

1	2	③	④	5	⑥	7	8	9	10

1. Starving and irritable; being this hungry is painful
2. Very hungry, uncomfortable, and loud rumblings in your stomach
3. Hungry; wanting to eat
4. Just a little hungry
5. Neither hungry nor full
6. Just at that point of fullness; perfectly content
7. Just beyond fullness; you've had enough but could find room for a few more bites
8. Uncomfortable; wish you hadn't had those last few bites; want to wear only loose clothing
9. Very uncomfortable and bloated
10. So full that it feels like Thanksgiving

Your notes might look something like this:

Before eating: ___3___

10 minutes into my meal: ___4___

After eating: ___6___

Think Before You Drink

It's easy to mindlessly sip extra calories. Nearly zero-calorie coffee and tea balloon to hundreds of calories if you add syrups and cream. A single can of soda or glass of sweet iced tea provides about 150 calories. Fruit juices also have lots of calories, so pay attention to your serving size. A 4-ounce glass of juice is the equivalent of a small piece of fruit. Alcohol provides a double whammy of calories because alcoholic beverages contain calories, plus they cause lots of us to lose our inhibitions and eat more food than we would otherwise. Some good beverage choices are these:

- Water
- Unsweetened tea and coffee
- Tomato and vegetable juice
- Small glass of 100% fruit juice
- Low-fat and nonfat milk and soymilk
- Unsweetened plain or flavored sparkling water or seltzer
- Seltzer water with a splash of your favorite fruit juice
- Water infused with your favorite flavors such as cucumber and mint or blueberries and lavender

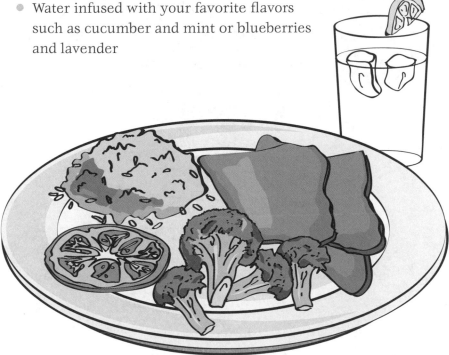

4 ounces lean roast beef: 200 calories

1 cup roasted broccoli prepared with olive oil: 71 calories

½ cup brown rice: 108 calories

Sliced tomato: 22 calories

Zero-calorie flavored seltzer: 0 calories

Total Calories: 401

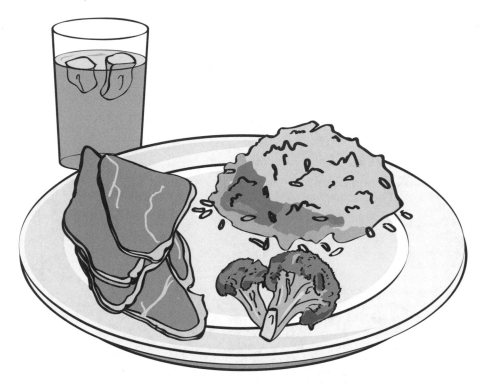

6 ounces mostly lean roast beef: 277 calories

½ cup roasted broccoli prepared with olive oil: 36 calories

1 cup brown rice: 216 calories

12-ounce glass of fruit punch: 195 calories

Total Calories: 724 calories

Monitoring Your Weight

For most people, I favor self-weighing. But it can have disastrous effects for some. If you stand on the scale and use the number—whatever that number is—as information and feedback to your weight control efforts, then weighing is a good idea. But if the number affects your mood and if it offers judgment instead of information, don't weigh yourself. The number on the scale cannot tell you a thing about your worthiness. It should not tell you that it's a good day when you like the number and that it's a bad day when you're displeased with the number. It's a number. That's all it is. Don't allow it to affect your self-esteem.

If you choose to weigh yourself, check the reliability of your scale. Stand on it three times without changing clothes, drinking water, or using the bathroom. Your scale is reliable enough if it gives the same number within 1 pound or so with each of the three tests. So if your scale weighs you at 177, 179, and 175, it's unreliable. Either purchase a more reliable scale or plan to weigh yourself at the gym or the doctor's office. Check your weight weekly or even more often. This way, you receive feedback for your plan and you can adjust your diet and exercise routine as necessary. But if the scale becomes a source of anxiety, weigh yourself less often or not at all. If you're trying to maintain your weight, I recommend weighing yourself very often, so you can catch small gains before they become unmanageable.

Some reasons your weight may be elevated

The most obvious reason is that you're eating more calories or burning fewer calories. But the obvious answer isn't always the right answer. Sometimes the reason your weight is up a pound or two overnight has nothing to do with gaining fat. Here are some other reasons:

1. *Your sodium intake is up.* If you've eaten out more than usual where high-sodium fare is the norm or had extra-salty meals at home, your body will hold more fluid.
2. *You added carbohydrates to a typical low-carb diet.* If your body is used to subsisting on a fairly low carb intake, eating more carbs causes more glycogen and water storage.
3. *You haven't had a bowel movement.*
4. *Hormonal changes.* A woman can expect to see a couple pounds of fluid changes because of her menstrual cycle.

Keep a Food Record

People who keep food records tend to lose more weight than people who don't keep food records. And those who keep the most food records lose the most weight. Recording your food choices increases your awareness and makes you accountable to yourself. Feel free to use a notebook, a journal designed for tracking food intake, a computer spreadsheet, or a smartphone app. Below is an example of a food record, and there is a blank template in Appendix B on page 273.

Today's goal: _Eat fruit and/or vegetable at each meal and snack_

Time/Meal (Place)	Food, Amount, Preparation	Notes
7:00 A.M./ Breakfast (Home)	Black coffee 1 cup low-fat cottage cheese, sprinkled with cinnamon, 1 tsp honey, 1/8 cup raisins	Started eating at a 4 on the Hunger Ruler. Finished at a 6.
10:00 A.M./ Snack (Office)	1/4 cup almonds	Regular break time
12:30 P.M./ Lunch (Break room)	Egg salad on lettuce (2 eggs, 1 Tbsp light mayo) 10 Triscuit Thin Crisps crackers 1 cup cherry tomatoes, 3 mini bell peppers 1 small clementine Can of no-calorie flavored seltzer water	Started eating at a 3 on the Hunger Ruler. Finished at a 6.
3:30 P.M./ Snack (Office)	Cup of unsweetened tea	
4:30 P.M./ Snack (Office)	Cup of unsweetened decaf green tea 1 medium apple	
7:00 P.M./ Dinner (Home)	1/2 cup brown rice, cooked in vegetable broth 1 cup black beans with onions and peppers 1/4 cup nonfat plain Greek yogurt and fresh herbs, on top of black beans and rice 1 cup steamed green beans, seasoned with olive oil (2 tsp) and garlic 1 cup 1% milk 4 chocolate kisses	Started eating at a 4 on the Hunger Ruler. Finished at a 7. Wanted more but brushed my teeth instead. ☺

Here are some tips to make the most of your food record.

- *Make it convenient.* Decide if you'll do better electronically or with old-fashioned paper and pencil. Regardless, your record needs to stay with you, so keep that in mind.
- *Identify what you need to record.* If you're trying to get a handle on emotional eating or mindless eating, you'll benefit from including your location, activities, and emotions when you eat. If you're tracking calories, add that to your food record. Make it easy on yourself by recording only what's important to you. For that matter, if you have breakfast and lunch under control, make notes for dinner and snacks only.
- *Record throughout the day.* If you keep track of your food as you are about to eat it or at least immediately after eating it, you have a chance at this meal or the next one to alter your behavior. On the other hand, if you sit down at the end of the day to report back what you ate, you've lost all opportunity for immediate feedback and a chance at rectifying poor decisions.
- *Be honest and thorough.* Sometimes people choose not to keep a food record on the days they don't eat according to plan. This practice is definitely unhelpful.
- *Record beverages and nibbles.* They add up. Once I helped a young mom identify that she was eating a few hundred calories extra every day by taking bites from her children's plates. Once she nixed that, she dropped 10 pounds pretty quickly.
- *Reflect daily.* Give your food record an honest appraisal daily, and use your assessment to set a SMART eating goal for tomorrow. Choose something that you want to continue to do well or something that you want to do better. In the example above, the writer set the goal to eat fruits, vegetables, or both at each meal and snack.
- *Reflect weekly or monthly.* Make note of the positive changes you've achieved over time. Take a few minutes to feel the pride. Then vow to continue.

Steer Clear of Dubious Weight Loss Programs

There is lots of money to be made in weight loss programs and supplements. Because of this, there are plenty of unscrupulous people selling unhelpful and potentially dangerous programs and products. Generally, if something sounds too good to be true, it probably is. In fact, one study found that herbal and dietary supplements cause about 20% of liver toxicity cases. Keep in mind that if there were easy ways to lose weight, very few people would be overweight. Both losing weight and keeping weight off are hard. Watch out for weight loss programs with these red flags:

- They tell you that diet and exercise don't matter. Or they say that calories don't count.
- They claim that the program or product works for everyone. They don't consider your preferences, health status, and individual needs.
- You're instructed to eliminate a large list of foods or whole food groups.
- The program comes with a long list of diet rules.
- They promise very large weight loss or very rapid weight loss.
- They tell you that the weight loss is permanent.
- The "proof" of success is based on before and after photos and testimonials from dieters.
- They use sensational words like "breakthrough," "secret formula," and "miraculous."
- The program is expensive, or they tell you that you must sign up right away because the price is about to increase.

Medical Weight Loss Treatments

If your risk for obesity-related health problems is very high, you may want to discuss various medical treatments with your health care provider.

Medications

There are several prescription weight loss medications available that help people lose weight when added to lifestyle changes. Most are pills that help suppress appetite. One drug (orlistat) inhibits fat digestion and absorption. Another weight loss medication (liraglutide) is a higher dose of a diabetes drug and is taken by injection. It keeps food in your stomach longer and helps you feel less hungry. Depending on the specific drug, participants in weight loss studies dropped an average of 4–14% of their starting weight after 1 year. While this is probably not enough to bring many people to their dream weights, this amount of weight loss is quite beneficial to health.

Weight Loss Surgery

Weight loss surgery, also called bariatric surgery or metabolic surgery, is a tool typically reserved for individuals with a BMI above 40 kg/m² or with a BMI above 30 kg/m² plus significant obesity-related health conditions or complications such as poorly controlled type 2 diabetes. There are different types of bariatric surgery, and each has a different average weight loss and different advantages and disadvantages. According to the Obesity Action Coalition, most people undergoing metabolic surgery will lose 10–35% of their presurgery weight within 2–3 years of the procedure. Some surgical procedures affect gut hormones that reduce appetite. Others do not. Even before much weight loss has occurred, some types of metabolic surgery result in better blood glucose control.

Weight Loss Devices

These devices are approved by the U.S. Food and Drug Administration to treat obesity.

- A gastric balloon is placed in the stomach to take up space and increase feelings of fullness with less food.

- A gastric emptying system involves placing a tube between the stomach and the outside of the abdomen to drain part of a meal after eating.

Each medication, type of surgery, and medical device comes with risks and potential side effects. Have a thoughtful conversation with your health care provider to ensure you make a wise and careful decision about the best treatment options for you.

Be Empowered

- Using the list on page 66, identify your motivators to lose weight.
- Select a reasonable weight loss goal.
- Identify a reasonable daily calorie range and at least three steps to achieve it.
- Create SMART goals around calorie-saving strategies.
- Keep a food record.
- If appropriate, initiate a conversation with your health care provider about medical weight loss strategies.

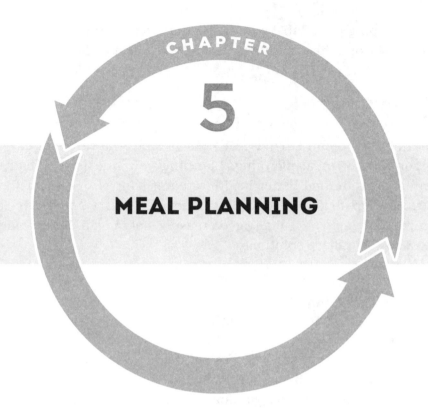

CHAPTER

5

MEAL PLANNING

*I*t is curious that some of the best planners neglect to plan their meals. Even people who use their planning skills successfully and habitually at work and in their personal lives often fail to plan what or when they will eat. I suppose it's because food is so readily available that it seems unnecessary to plan. Also, many people think that healthful eating is more about willpower than anything else. I assure you that willpower has very little to do with healthful eating and that planning has quite a lot to do with it. As we've already discussed, willpower is little more than magical thinking, and the myth of willpower is the undoing of many good intentions.

Every time you eat or drink is an opportunity. What you eat in the short term affects your energy level, feelings of comfort or discomfort, and perhaps your mood and ability to do work. What you eat over time affects your long-term well-being, including your risks of developing type 2 diabetes, dementia, and other chronic health problems. Something this important deserves some planning.

Common Barriers to Meal Planning

The most common barrier I've seen is lack of awareness of the importance of meal planning. Planning your meals can lead to better nutrition and better health, greater control over your food choices, more food variety, saving money, less waste, and much less stress. But people have many good reasons not to plan. Fortunately, most obstacles have solutions.

- *It takes time.* Yes, it does take time upfront, but it's worth it. And in the long term, it will probably save time. Once you have experience with meal planning, you can re-use older menu plans.
- *It's hard to please everyone.* It's helpful to give everyone a say in the menu. Family members can take turns picking entrees and sides. If you have picky diners, pair less favorable foods with favorite foods, so everyone has something to eat and like. And remember not to pressure anyone to eat foods they don't like. Food acceptance increases with exposure, not pressure.
- *Family members have conflicting schedules.* With my kids involved in after-school sports and jobs, this happened to my family quite a lot. It helped to factor schedules into the plan. Some planned meals were nothing more than leftovers or soup and sandwiches. Or often I used my slow cooker, so I could serve dinner in that tiny window of opportunity. And sometimes that window was mighty tiny! What saved us from unhealthful eating was the plan. It's okay to plan something as simple as a sandwich.
- *There are too many surprises in your week.* Have a backup meal plan. By stocking your pantry, refrigerator, and freezer smartly, you can always whip up something quickly. Scrambled eggs,

frozen vegetables, and potatoes are delicious and far more wholesome than a bucket of greasy chicken.

- *You don't know what a healthful meal looks like.* Review the section of healthful eating patterns in Chapter 3. Give a close look at the Plate Method of meal planning on page 52. And check out the menu ideas at the end of Chapter 6 on page 168.
- *You don't know what to cook.* Start a collection of go-to recipes and meals. First include your family favorites. Then add more by searching the Internet. A few terrific websites are the American Diabetes Association's My Food Advisor® (http://tracker.diabetes.org), Cooking Light (http://www.cookinglight.com), and EatingWell (http://www.eatingwell.com). Keep reading for more menu ideas.

Two Methods of Meal Planning

If you are new to meal planning, you may prefer a very detailed and structured method. If all you need is a little organization, try the mix-and-match method.

Detailed Meal Planning

1. *Look ahead.* This is the critical step that many people skip. Look at your calendar and, if applicable, talk to your family to learn about schedules and other obstacles to a planned dinner. Consider if you have a late appointment, sports activities for your kids, or some other activity that cuts into your meal preparation time. If you do, choose a meal that's quick to make like sandwiches, tuna salad, or leftovers.
2. *Put your plan on paper.* Jot down full dinners that you plan to serve your family. Use a calendar or one of the templates in Appendix B. The Detailed Weekly Menu Planner template (page 274) has room for breakfast, lunch, and dinner. Fill in each

meal or just those with which you need extra help. The *Plate Method* dinner template guides you to plan a meat or vegetarian entrée, a starchy food, and one or more non-starchy vegetables. Many people like putting their planned meals on a dry-erase board that hangs in their kitchens. Whatever method you choose—paper, dry-erase, or electronic calendar—simply write in each food you plan to serve.

- Decide which dinner meals need to be quick-to-prepare foods or leftovers and which meals can be put together more leisurely.
- Using your family's favorite meals, your recipe collection, and ideas for quick meals, start filling in the blanks. Don't forget to plan for leftovers, either for another dinner or for lunches. It saves times to cook once to eat twice. For example, you might prepare salmon, quinoa, and roasted broccoli for dinner and serve salmon salad later in the week.

If you're new to meal planning, make it easy on yourself and start with your favorite recipes and menu ideas. Continue this process with lunches and breakfasts or stick with dinner only. If you have lunches and breakfasts down pat, don't waste your effort adding them to your meal plan. Or if the process is overwhelming, start with dinner and move to other meals when you feel more confident or energized.

3. *Take inventory.* Add any ingredients or staple items that you don't have on hand to your grocery list.
4. *Build flexibility into your plan.* If an item is on special at the grocery store or if you simply have a desire to try something new, go for it. A plan is your guide, not a set of rules that you must follow. Make it work for you by remaining flexible.
5. *Recycle your menus.* Make everything as easy on yourself as possible. Without allowing yourself to get into a food rut, reuse what works. Keep your menus in a paper folder or on your computer. After you have 3 or 4 weeks of menus, take the best of each to create the next one.

Mix-and-Match Meal Planning

If too much structure gets you down or if you're already practiced with meal planning, use this flexible method as your guide. I've been doing this for years. A Mix-and-Match Weekly Menu Planner template is in Appendix B on page 279.

1. *Look ahead.* Again, don't ignore this critical step. Without knowing what might get in the way of putting a healthful meal on the table, you're leaving yourself open to choosing meals that are too complicated for the time you have available and wasting food you're not able to prepare.

2. *Select entrees and side dishes.* If your review of the week ahead tells you, for example, that you'll need six dinners, choose six entrees, six nonstarchy vegetables, and six starchy foods. You don't need to plan each meal in full, just be sure to have enough food planned for each category. That's the mix-and-match part of this. Your starch category might include roasted potatoes, canned corn, quinoa, brown rice, and sweet potatoes. You can decide shortly before cooking which entrée and nonstarchy vegetable to match them with.

3. *Take inventory.* Identify which ingredients you have on hand, and add everything else to your grocery list. Don't feel compelled to preselect each item, especially vegetables. As long as you know the proper number for each category, you can decide in the supermarket based on availability and affordability.

4. *Fill in the rest of the meals.* In a similar manner, decide how many lunches you'll eat at home and how many you will pack. Select the required number of fruits, vegetables, sandwich meats, etc. Add the necessary items to your list. Do the same for the foods you will need for breakfasts and snacks.

Go-To Meals

You probably already have a handful of favorite meals to prepare when you have the luxury of time and other go-to meals for when time is tight. Putting them in print now will help you when you're meal planning. It's also helpful to have backup meal ideas when your original plan won't work. So add some ideas for wholesome foods that you can prepare quickly or pick up when necessary. There are several suggestions below.

Planned Backup Meals

What would you prepare for dinner if the chicken you intended to cook was spoiled or if you returned home too late to cook it? And what would you eat for lunch at work if you accidently left your packed lunch at home? You can see that eating healthfully in these situations has less to do with willpower and discipline and more to do with skills, strategies, and plans. The following ideas can serve as inspiration.

At home:

- Scrambled eggs, ready-to-heat brown rice, frozen vegetable
- Tuna salad, whole-grain crackers, canned or fresh fruit
- Low-fat cottage cheese topped with fruit and nuts or diced tomatoes and basil; serve with toast or crackers
- Bean burrito made by mixing the following canned items together: drained kidney beans, drained tomatoes, fat-free refried beans, diced green chiles, and diced black olives; mix in reduced-fat shredded cheese and heat. Serve with whole-grain tortillas, nonfat Greek yogurt or sour cream, and jarred salsa. To keep the sodium in check, use no-salt-added varieties of canned products or mix no-salt-added varieties and regular varieties.
- Panini made with whole-grain bread, reduced-fat cheese, sliced vegetables or fruit. Serve with bagged salad or prepared vegetable soup.

- Rotisserie chicken, baked potatoes, frozen or canned vegetables
- Steamed shrimp, ready-to-heat brown rice or quinoa, canned or frozen vegetable

At work:

- Frozen or shelf-stable meal. See page 113 for nutrition guidelines.
- Liquid meal replacement. Look for one with at least 10 grams protein, but 20 grams is better, and no more than 3 grams saturated fat.
- Tuna or salmon from ready-to-serve pouches or easy-to-open cans and whole-grain crackers
- Whole-grain bread or crackers with peanut butter or almond butter

Plan for Snacks

Over the last few decades snacking has become a bit of a national pastime. We consume a few hundred more calories now than we did in the late 1970s, and most of the additional calories are eaten between meals. In fact, on average, we consume about one-quarter of our total calories as snacks. This makes planning for snacks as critical as planning for meals.

You may have heard that you should graze or snack often to rev your metabolism or to lose weight. This is one of those common pieces of advice that is inconsistent with current science. As discussed in Chapter 4 under Metabolic Rate, the thermic effect of food, or TEF (the extra calories burned to process food and nutrients), is not related to the frequency of eating, but is related to the type and amount of food you eat. The short story is, that over a full day, your metabolic rate will not differ if you eat the exact same foods in many small meals or fewer larger meals. Some people find that eating more often helps with appetite control, and others find that snacking often does little more than add calories to their total intake.

Research studies also find various results, and experts say that there is no ideal eating frequency for weight control, blood glucose management, and cholesterol management.

To Snack or Not To Snack?

Whether or not noshing between meals is good for you depends on you. Do you like to snack? Does it help you manage your hunger? Does it fit into your day? Does it contribute to a nutritious diet?

- Enjoy a planned snack if it helps you tame appetite and rein in out-of-control eating later on. A piece of fruit on your afternoon commute, for example, may keep you from raiding the refrigerator when you get home, or it may help prevent overeating at dinner.
- Don't snack to boost your metabolic rate. It doesn't help.
- Snack when you're hungry and a meal is more than a short time away. Don't panic though. Regardless of what you've heard, being hungry doesn't mean that you're starving, wasting muscle, digesting your stomach lining, or suffering blood glucose swings. It simply means that you haven't eaten for a while.
- Don't snack because others are eating, because you're bored, or because it's your habit.
- Eat a planned snack to fit in wholesome foods. Ask yourself what you're not getting enough of at meals. The answer is probably a good snack choice.
- Snack if you need to fuel a workout or replenish after a hard workout. There's often no need to snack before or after a light or short workout.

Healthful Snacks

If snacking is right for you, identify healthful, tasty snacks to satisfy your hunger. It's a good idea to keep a written list to avoid the mental drain of weighing options and relying on willpower every time you want a snack. Keep the list in your smartphone or on the refrigerator, kitchen counter, desk, or wherever it is that you will snack. Write down the appropriate portion size, and if you are counting calories, include that, too. Unless you are very active, your snacks should probably range from 100 to 250 calories each. Below are a few ideas, but the best ideas will probably be your own.

- Any fresh, frozen, canned, or dried fruit, preferably without added sugars
- 1/2 peanut butter sandwich on whole-grain bread
- Apple and peanut butter or almond butter
- 1 ounce of nuts, about 1/4 cup
- Fruit and nuts, such as a small pear and 1/8 cup walnuts
- Hummus with raw vegetables such as cucumber, cauliflower, bell peppers, and carrots
- Hummus and whole-grain crackers
- Strained yogurt (Greek or Icelandic) with fresh or frozen berries
- Low-fat cottage cheese with diced tomatoes, black pepper, and fresh basil leaves
- Low-fat cottage cheese and fruit
- 3–5 cups light popcorn
- Reduced-fat cheese and apple slices or grapes
- Vegetable juice or tomato juice with almonds or reduced-fat cheese
- Hard-boiled egg and whole-grain crackers
- Mashed hard-boiled egg on cucumber rounds
- 1 ounce roasted chickpeas and 1/8 cup dried fruit
- Snack bar of primarily whole grains or fruit or both whole grains and fruit

Be Empowered

- Write a list of three to five backup dinners. Add pantry and freezer staples to your shopping list.
- If you work away from home, create a list of foods to keep handy when you need a snack or lunch. Add them to your shopping list.
- Create your personal snack menu. Add any necessary items to your shopping list.
- Start or add to your recipe collection.
- Experiment with at least one of the menu-planning templates in Appendix B.

CHAPTER

6

SHOPPING FOR GROCERIES AND PREPARING MEALS

*N*ow that you're on your way to planning your meals, you need to purchase wholesome food and prepare it in wholesome ways. Fortunately, there are a lot of tasty tweaks to make recipes more nourishing. Unfortunately, there are a lot of traps in the supermarket that might have you giving in to temptation or purchasing food that's only masquerading as healthful.

Savvy Supermarket Shopping

If you have fallen for these health traps, you're not alone. Supermarkets are overwhelming, and grocery shopping is not always tons of fun. Here are five pieces of bad advice.

- *Bad advice #1: Shop only the perimeter of the store.* The outside aisles of the store are home to plenty of not-so-healthful choices including baked goods, hot dogs, and ice cream. And if you skip the inside aisles, you'll miss a slew of wholesome items such as canned beans, vegetables, fruits, and tuna; whole grains like farro and brown rice; whole-grain breads and cereals; spices; tea bags; and nuts and nut butters.
- *Bad advice #2: Avoid processed foods.* This soundbite is much too broad to be useful. Toaster pastries are processed, and I don't recommend adding them to your shopping list. But canned beans and tuna are also processed. So are cartons of vegetable broth and quick-cooking brown rice. These are health-boosting processed foods that can make getting a nutritious meal on the table easier, faster, and less expensive. Let's not put toaster pastries and bologna in the same category as quick-cooking oats and canned salmon.
- *Bad advice #3: Choose only foods labeled natural or organic.* Unfortunately, *natural* doesn't have a legal definition (at least not yet), but the U.S. Food and Drug Administration (FDA) is considering one. *Organic* has a lengthy legal definition, but even that is no guarantee of wholesomeness. An organic cookie (regardless of the type of sugar used) is still a cookie and should be eaten in moderation. And if the price of organic produce prevents you from eating ample fruits and vegetables, your diet is much worse off than if you ate the less expensive conventional fruits and vegetables.
- *Bad advice #4: When in doubt, choose the one without.* We touched on this in Chapter 3, but it's important enough to mention again. Claims like fat-free, gluten-free, no cholesterol, no added sugar, and dairy-free seem to be on more packages than ever. Labels like these have the potential to confuse shoppers into thinking that a packaged food lacking an ingredient is more healthful than another packaged food with the ingredient. That just isn't true. For example, unless you have a gluten

intolerance, there's no reason to avoid gluten. And choosing a gluten-free product often means choosing the one with more sodium; added sugar, calories, or saturated fat; and less vitamins and minerals. Putting emphasis on what is missing distracts us from what is present—basically vitamins, minerals, fiber, and other under-consumed nutrients. Putting strict avoidance on an ingredient can also lead you astray by causing you to miss out on some nutrient-rich foods. There's nothing wrong with small amounts of added sugars, if a little sweetness helps you to eat health-shielding foods. If manufacturers didn't add sugar to dried cranberries and tart cherries, few people would eat them and benefit from their disease-fighting phytonutrients.

- *Bad advice #5: Skip anything with more than five ingredients.* The number of ingredients has nothing to do with the nutritional value of a food. What those ingredients are has quite a bit to do with nutrition, though. A quick lunch of packaged black bean or lentil soup with its 10 or more ingredients is a pretty good choice when those ingredients are beans, vegetables, herbs, spices, and cooking oil. A better strategy is to look at the ingredients to see if they are ones you can feel good about.

And here are seven tips to make your shopping more efficient and healthy:

1. *Shop with a list.* If you can, prepare your list according to the layout of your store. You'll shop faster and avoid some impulse buys.
2. *Carry a handbasket.* If you need just a few items, pick up a handbasket, so you can't load up a cart with tempting foods you don't need.
3. *Read the fine print.* Skip the bold letter front of package claims and head straight to the back to carefully read the Nutrition Facts panel and ingredients list.

4. *Avoid foods with partially hydrogenated oils.* If you see this ingredient, there is at least a trace amount of unhealthful trans fats present. The FDA will no longer allow manufacturers to use these unhealthful oils beginning in June 2018.

5. *Ignore "made with" claims.* The unanswered question is, "Made with how much?" Many packages tout *made with whole grains* or *made with real fruit,* but it could be just a pinch of whole grains mixed with a lot of refined grains or just a dot of real fruit mixed with a lot of added sugars and colors.

6. *Beware of "specials."* Usually, you don't need to buy the full amount advertised for a special. A sign may read "5 for $5," but you can often buy just one for a dollar. Keep in mind, too, that often the specials are for items that we don't need. If that's the case, leave the food in the store.

7. *Check before checking out.* Double-check your list to be sure that you've picked up everything you need. Equally important is to give a final review for each item in your cart that's not on your list. Ask yourself if those foods are going to help or hurt your healthful eating plan.

Reading a Food Label

Deciphering food labels is one of those skills that is more complicated than it seems.

Ingredients List

Ingredients are listed by quantity. The first ingredient identified is the one that is present in the greatest amount. Look over the ingredients to avoid anything to which you may be allergic or intolerant. There may be many sources of added sugars or sodium. You do not need to identify each source of sodium because the total is listed on the Nutrition Facts panel. As manufacturers roll out the new labels,

Serving Size: Look here first because everything on the label is for this amount of food. In this example, you could measure out ½ cup of this food using measuring cups or 40 grams by using a food scale. Don't confuse serving size with recommended portion size. Some serving sizes have recently changed to reflect the amount that people have been eating. In recent years, people have been serving up larger amounts of ice cream than in decades past. So now, the serving size on a tub of ice cream is larger than ½ cup. That doesn't mean, though, that you should eat more than ½ cup.

Calories: If weight is your concern, the calorie line is what you want to look at. Ask yourself how one serving (or more) would fit into your total calorie allowance.

Cholesterol: The blood cholesterol levels of some—but not most—people are greatly affected by the cholesterol in food. It's prudent to limit dietary cholesterol, but keeping a lid on the amounts of saturated and trans fats is far more important.

Saturated Fat and Trans Fat: These fats are harmful to the heart, and they likely make you less sensitive to insulin. Limit saturated fats and avoid all trans fats.

Polyunsaturated Fat and Monounsaturated Fat: These heart-healthy fats improve insulin resistance when they are consumed in place of saturated fats. The FDA does not require that they are listed on food labels, but when you subtract the amount of saturated and trans fats from the total fat listed, you are left with unsaturated fat. It's up to manufacturers whether or not to include polyunsaturated and monounsaturated fats on food labels.

Sodium: Limit sodium to keep blood pressure in check.

Total Carbohydrate: This includes starch, naturally occurring sugar, added sugar, fiber, and sugar alcohol. The FDA does not require that each category of carbohydrate be listed on a food label.

Fiber: There are many types of fibers with various functions, including colon health, blood sugar management, and cholesterol lowering. It's important to eat many types of fiber-containing foods.

Total Sugars: This number includes both naturally occurring sugars found in milk, fruit, vegetables, and other foods as well as sugars that are added during processing.

Added sugars: Limit these to meet your nutrient needs while controlling your calorie intake. Added sugars include syrups like honey and agave nectar too.

% Daily Value: This number tells you how much one serving of food contributes to a total amount that's recommended for an average 2000-calorie diet. Your own diet may be more or fewer calories, however. In this sample label, one serving of food provides 20% of the recommended minimum intake for calcium, 5% of the recommended maximum intake for saturated fat, and 14% of the recommended minimum intake for fiber. The % DV is useful when comparing two or more products.

Nutrition Facts

8 servings per container

Serving size   1/2 cup (40g)

Amount per serving

Calories   230

	% Daily Value*
Total Fat 8g	**10%**
Saturated Fat 1g	**5%**
Trans Fat 0g	
Polyunsaturated Fat 4g	
Monounsaturated Fat 3g	
Cholesterol 0mg	**0%**
Sodium 280mg	**12%**
Total Carbohydrate 37g	**13%**
Dietary Fiber 4g	**14%**
Total Sugars 13g	
Includes 10g Added Sugars	**20%**
Protein 7g	
Vitamin D 2mcg	10%
Calcium 260mg	20%
Iron 1mg	6%
Potassium 235mg	6%

* The % Daily Value (DV) tells you how much a nutrient in a serving of food contributes to a daily diet. 2,000 calories a day is used for general nutrition advice.

the total amount of added sugars will also be easy to find on the Nutrition Facts panel.

Shopping by the Aisles

A lot of people dislike grocery shopping. These tips for each section of the supermarket should help you make it a better experience and have you bringing home the best of each aisle.

Produce Section

Because vegetables and fruits should make up a large part of your diet, they should fill up your shopping cart, too. Most adults should aim for 1 1/2 to 2 cups of fruits and 2–3 cups of vegetables each day. Sadly, as a nation, we consume only 59% of the recommended amount of vegetables and 42% of our target fruit intake. Feel free to buy and eat a variety of fresh, dried, frozen, and canned fruits and vegetables. To get the most out of the produce section, you'll need to shop regularly—at least weekly.

Many people ask what are the best or most healthful fruits and vegetables. Although some experts have tried to create a list, it's really a question that has no good answer. Because each fruit and vegetable holds a unique array of nutrients and phytonutrients, our best nutrition comes from eating a large variety in ample amounts.

- Aim for every color
  - Green: kiwi, grapes, bell pepper, celery, broccoli, avocado
  - Red: cherries, watermelon, radish, tomato, bell pepper
  - White/brown: banana, apple, pear, cauliflower, mushrooms, onion
  - Yellow/orange: apricot, peach, orange, pineapple, bell pepper, carrots
  - Blue/purple: plum, blueberries, blackberries, cabbage, purple onion

- Aim for a variety of types
  - Melon: cantaloupe, watermelon
  - Berries: strawberries, blueberries, raspberries
  - Stone fruits (also called drupes): apricots, plums, nectarines, cherries
  - Pomes: apples, pears
  - Citrus: orange, grapefruit, clementine
  - Cruciferous vegetables: broccoli, cabbage, cauliflower
  - Leafy greens: arugula, spinach, lettuce, kale
  - Root vegetables: carrots, beets, radishes, turnips, parsnips
  - Starchy vegetables: white potatoes, sweet potatoes, corn, peas
- Buy produce at varying degrees of ripeness. If you and your family are fond of avocados and bananas, for example, pick up some ripe ones to eat now and under-ripe ones for later in the week.
- Pick up a few fresh herbs to liven up your meals.
- For convenience, buy ready-to-eat or ready-to-cook vegetables and salad greens.
- Buy the amount you truly need. You don't need to purchase a bunch of bananas if you want only one or two. And you rarely need to purchase the full bag of grapes, cherries, and other produce packaged in open bags. As long as these items are sold by weight, simply pluck out the amount you want. If you want a very small amount of produce, make your selection from the supermarket's salad bar. Store what you buy in sealed bags or containers in your refrigerator until you're ready to cook it.

Dairy Case and Other Refrigerated Items

This area of the grocery store can be a calorie, saturated fat, and added sugar landmine. In general, you are better off looking for non-fat and low-fat dairy choices. These options are lower in calories (there are 150 calories in 1 cup of whole milk but 90 calories in 1 cup

They're Filling, Low-Calorie, Nutritious, and Come in Lots of Varieties!

Yes, I'm talking about nonstarchy vegetables. They provide fewer calories than an equivalent amount of other foods—about 25 calories per 1/2 cup cooked vegetables or 1 cup raw vegetables. For this reason (and many others), I encourage you eat them throughout the day and not just at dinner. Take a look at this list of nonstarchy vegetables to see what a huge variety is available. And this is not even a complete list!

Artichoke and artichoke hearts	Jicama
Asparagus	Kale
Bamboo shoots	Kohlrabi
Beans (green beans and wax beans)	Lettuce and salad greens (arugula, butterhead, endive, frisee, radicchio, romaine, mache, iceberg, escarole, looseleaf)
Beets	Mushrooms (white, cremini, oyster, portabello, shiitake, enoki)
Broccoli	Okra
Brussels sprouts	Onions (red, white, yellow, leeks, scallions)
Cabbage (green, red, bok choy)	Pea pods
Carrots	Peppers
Cauliflower	Radishes
Celery	Rutabaga
Cucumber	Spinach
Daikon	Sugar snap peas
Eggplant	Summer squash (yellow, pattypan, zucchini)
Fennel	Swiss chard
Gourds (bitter melon, luffa)	Tomatoes
Greens (collards, dandelion, mustard, purslane, turnip)	Turnips
Heart of palm	Water chestnuts

of nonfat milk) and provide less saturated fat. Some research suggests that dairy fat is less harmful than other saturated fats and some suggests that dairy fat is even beneficial. For now, because of the preponderance of the scientific evidence, major health organizations like the American Diabetes Association and the American Heart Association still recommend limiting saturated fats from all types of food. If you have a favorite whole-milk dairy food such as cheddar cheese or yogurt, eat it in small quantities and choose larger portions of other dairy foods in their lower-fat versions. To limit added sugars, choose plain yogurt, milk, and cottage cheese and review the Nutrition Facts label to select brands and varieties with only small amounts of added sugars. Flavored milk and yogurt may also be sweetened with artificial sweeteners.

- *Milk:* Cow's milk and soymilk are the only ones that provide a good dose of protein. If you like the taste of almond milk or other plant-based milk, they are fine to use in recipes and as a flavored beverage. Just don't expect them to be the nutritional equivalent of cow's milk.
- *Yogurt and drinkable yogurt:* Yogurt is made when live bacteria cultures ferment milk. Some yogurts are later heat-treated, killing the beneficial microbes. To identify yogurt with probiotics, look for the words *live active cultures* on the label. Choose lower-calorie and lower-added-sugar products. Strained varieties like Greek and Icelandic yogurt tend to be higher in protein and lower in carbohydrate (lactose) than traditional yogurt, but both kinds are nutrient dense. Because it is thicker, plain strained yogurt expertly replaces sour cream in dips and as a chili or baked potato topping.
- *Cheese:* Reduced-fat cheeses have come a long way from the days of those plastic-like slices that wouldn't melt. You should find ample tasty and meltable varieties of 50% reduced-fat cheese and some even as much as 75% reduced-fat. When choosing full-fat cheeses, opt for strongly flavored ones like

sharp cheddar, blue cheese, and feta to get a big flavor punch in a small amount.

- *Butter and spreads:* Use butter only now and then when other options just won't do. A pat of butter here and there is just fine, but tablespoon after tablespoon is not. Spreadable butter-like options are more healthful choices. Look for one made with a liquid vegetable oil and with as little saturated fat as possible, and no more than 3 grams saturated fat per tablespoon. While coconut oil may be a suitable option for baking, it's far too high in unhealthful saturated fats to be used often.

- *Eggs:* Eggs are one of only a few foods that are rich in cholesterol and low in saturated fats. Today we know that saturated fats are the bigger culprit in high blood cholesterol levels. However, this doesn't mean that very high intakes of cholesterol are okay. Eggs are a good source of protein and several other nutrients, so feel good about eating an egg or two. There are many types of eggs on the shelves, all of which are good choices. If you're not planning to fully cook your egg (like a poached or soft boiled egg), the federal government advises buying pasteurized eggs, which have been treated in a hot water bath to destroy illness-causing microbes.

- *Dips:* Making your own dips is often a good idea, but there are still some good choices to be found in the supermarket. Hummus is one of those. Carefully reading food labels will help you find others.

Deli Case

There's no need to avoid the deli case. It can be a terrific option for getting a quick sandwich or no-fuss dinner together.

- Sandwich meats vary significantly in nutritional quality. Two brands of lean turkey breast may have very different ingredients lists. Look for a product that contains meat and spices

Sugar or Alternative Sweeteners?

When you read food labels, you'll notice that quite a lot of foods contain added sugars. You'll find them in breads, yogurt, cereal, and peanut butter, in addition to the usual suspects like ice cream, cookies, and candy. A lot of people wonder if it's better to use artificial or nonnutritive sweeteners instead of added sugars. Many people worry about making a safe choice. I think that either choice is fine—if the amount you use is small. The American Diabetes Association, FDA, and other health organizations have found artificial and nonnutritive sweeteners are generally safe. Additionally, a little sugar in a nutrient-dense food like yogurt is unlikely to hurt you. But if you consume sugary drinks or foods several times daily, then you will surely get too many calories or too few nutrients, or both. Artificial or nonnutritive sweeteners can take the place of sugar in some of your beverages and foods, but they will help you lose weight only if you cut calories at the same time. Small amounts of either added sugars or alternative sweeteners can fit into a health-boosting, wholesome diet.

only. Avoid meats with fillers that dilute the protein and other nutrients while offering little to the taste and texture.

- Sodium runs high at the deli counter. Look for lower-sodium products, which are frequently still as much as 300–400 mg sodium per serving.
- Limit ham, bologna, salami, hot dogs, sausage, and other highly processed meats because they are linked to an increased risk of colon cancer.
- A few lighter cheese options are light Havarti, Jarlsberg light, and Alpine Lace Swiss.
- A rotisserie chicken is a good option to get dinner on the table quickly. Just keep in mind that the sodium is likely quite high, so balance your meal with lower-sodium sides.

- Unless the nutrition information is available for salads and other sides, it's best to skip them or limit them. Traditional macaroni salad, ambrosia, and others often have several hundred calories in a large serving. A few good options (but still watch your portion sizes) are bean salads, vinaigrette-based vegetable salads, and whole grain–based salads like those made with wild rice or quinoa.

Meat and Fish

When it comes to red meats and poultry, lean is king because the saturated fats in fatty meats are linked to both insulin resistance and heart disease. Fish is another story. Fatty fish are known to be a heart-healthy choice because they contain omega-3 fatty acids.

- The leanest cuts of beef have *loin* or *round* in the name, such as tenderloin and eye of round. The leanest cuts of pork have *loin* in their name.
- Buy only skinless poultry or dump the skin at home (before or after cooking) to save half the fat. But don't feel that you are stuck with white meat only. Although somewhat higher in calories and saturated fat, chicken and turkey thighs are still nutritious choices.
- Choose ground meat that is at least 90% lean. Usually 90–96% lean works well in tacos, spaghetti sauce, and the like. Read labels for ground turkey also because turkey is often ground with the skin, which adds extra fat.
- All fish and other seafood are good choices. Pregnant women, breast-feeding women, women who might get pregnant, and children should limit albacore tuna and avoid fish that is highest in mercury: tilefish from the Gulf of Mexico, shark, swordfish, and king mackerel. Most often, choose fish rich in omega-3 fatty acids, which includes salmon, trout, bluefish, herring, halibut, sardines, and tuna.

Freezer Aisle

Stock up on wholesome freezer items when the price is right.

- Keep a few healthful frozen meals on hand for when you need a quick lunch or dinner. Use the following as a general guide.
    - No more than 500 calories (400 or so for weight loss)
    - No more than 3 grams of saturated fat
    - 0 grams of trans fat
    - No more than 600 mg of sodium, but preferably less than 480 mg
    - At least 3 grams of fiber, but preferably 5 grams or more
    - At least 14 grams of protein, but preferably 25 grams or more
- Enjoy a wide variety of frozen fruits. The ingredients list should have fruit only. Smoothies are thicker and creamier when made with frozen fruit instead of fresh fruit and ice. Berries, grapes, bananas, and others straight out of the freezer make a tasty dessert or cooling snack, too.
- Keep several types of frozen vegetables on hand, since they are as nutritious and sometimes even more nutritious than fresh options. Vegetables should be the only ingredients. Heat them for a quick addition to your meal. Add them to soups and stews or mix them with whole grains for a hearty, nourishing side dish.
- Frozen shrimp and individually wrapped fish fillets defrost quickly under running water, and using these items can help you get a meal together quickly.
- When choosing ice cream and other frozen desserts, it's smart to buy items in individual servings. Try popsicles, ice cream bars, ice cream sandwiches, and individual slices of pie or cake. Read labels carefully to make sure these treat foods fit your health goals.

Breads

Whether it's sandwich bread, a pita for scooping hummus, or an English muffin for breakfast, most of your breads should be made of whole grains. Head straight to the ingredients list. Ideally, you will see whole wheat, whole oats, whole barley, brown rice, or other whole grain as the first ingredient. Enriched wheat flour is just another way to say white flour. Another way to identify whole grains is to look for the Whole Grain Council's yellow-gold Whole Grain Stamp on the front of the package. One version of the stamp identifies products that are 100% whole grain. A second version identifies products that contain at least one-half serving (8 grams) of whole grains.

- Don't let color confuse you. Some breads are brown because of molasses or coloring. And some light-colored breads are made of white whole-wheat flour, which has many of the same nutrients as other whole-wheat flour. White whole-wheat bread, however, does not have the same phytonutrients as traditional whole-wheat bread. Still, it's a wholesome choice, especially for people who prefer softer breads.
- Look for small rolls, pita breads, sandwich bread, tortillas, and bagels, particularly if you're watching your weight. A reasonable serving is 1 ounce, and you should be able to find ample choices for 70–90 calories per 1-ounce serving. Be cautious when selecting bagels. Even small ones can be more than 3 ounces, and large bagels could weigh as much as 5 ounces— the equivalent of 5 slices of bread.
- There are no hard and fast rules for choosing breads, but a good rule of thumb is to select products with at least 1 gram of fiber for every 50 calories. Even more fiber is better.

Crackers, Cereals, and Packaged Snacks

Use the same guidelines as above for selecting whole-grain products. And again, look for at least 1 gram of fiber for every 50 calories. If your cereal has 150 or so calories in a serving, it's good to have at least 3 grams of fiber.

- When comparing various flavors or brands, be sure to take note of the serving sizes. They may not be the same.
- Choose brands with fewer grams of *added* sugars. You'll find this information on the Nutrition Facts panel on the new food labels.
- Quick-cooking or long-cooking hot cereals are typically a better choice than instant hot cereals because the instant varieties tend to be much higher in sodium.
- Be on the lookout for junk food masquerading as healthful. A "breakfast cookie" is usually just a cookie with a bit more fiber or vitamins. Depending on how they're made, kale chips might top the scale on sodium and saturated fat. And cereal bars made with real fruit might actually contain more added sugars and flavors than real fruit.
- A few good choices in the snack aisle are nuts; dehydrated beet chips; roasted chickpeas; popcorn; whole-grain crackers; fruit leather made of 100% fruit; dried fruit; bars made of whole grains, dried fruit, nuts, and spices and little or no added sugars; and chips in 1-ounce packages.

Packaged and Canned Foods

Despite their bad reputation, canned foods are not necessarily overly processed or unhealthful. In fact, canned and other packaged foods can be quite wholesome and helpful in preparing tasty, convenient, affordable, and speedy meals. I've known people to avoid packaged groceries only to rely on less healthful fast food and other takeout when they're short on time. Use the same guidelines described for other types of groceries: carefully review serving size and calories; compare brands for sodium, saturated fat, and other nutrients of concern; and generally, select items that more closely resemble their natural state. If your family isn't ready for all no-salt-added canned goods, ease them slowly toward less sodium. Combine packages of regular canned vegetables with one without added salt. The result is much less sodium without much notice.

- *Beans:* Keep these on hand for stews, soups, and salads. If buying beans with added sodium, drain and rinse them before use to wash away about 40% of the sodium.
- *Lentils:* You might find bags of uncooked lentils near canned and uncooked dry beans, or your store may keep them near the rice and other grains. Uncooked lentils are a type of fast food. Unlike dried beans, they don't need to be soaked before cooking. Plus they cook fairly quickly. Red lentils can make it to the table in as little as 15 minutes. Green and brown lentils may cook for as long as 45 minutes. All lentils are powerhouses of nutrition. They give us resistant starches, fiber, vitamins, minerals, phytonutrients, and plant proteins. For extra ease, look for canned lentils.
- *Fish and other meats:* Make a quick sandwich or salad with tuna and salmon in cans or sealed pouches. To get a little extra calcium, choose salmon with the bones. To limit mercury (see page 112), opt for light tuna more often than albacore tuna. Feel free to select tuna packed in water or in oil. You'll likely use less mayonnaise or other binder if your tuna is oil-packed. Sardines are another good choice to add to salads or to place on top of crackers. Canned chicken is convenient as well, although it tends to have additives that may affect flavor and texture in desirable or undesirable ways. If you prefer to keep chicken on hand for those times when you need an impromptu speedy meal, canned chicken will serve you well. If you have the time to stop at the store, a rotisserie chicken is also a good option.
- *Tomatoes and tomato sauce:* Tomatoes are so versatile! Use them in soups, stews, casseroles, pasta dishes, and with beans, lentils,

chicken, fish, beef, and more. Try mixing up lower-sodium and regular products.

- *Tomato paste in a tube:* These handy tubes deliver as little or as much as your recipe requires. Once opened, store them in your refrigerator until next time. This product is terrific when you are eating more vegetarian meals because tomato paste provides a strong meaty flavor to beans and other vegetables.
- *Vegetables:* Canned green beans, jarred roasted bell peppers, and marinated artichoke hearts are just a few options. Buy canned vegetables for a side dish, to add to recipes, and for salads and sandwiches.
- *Fruits:* No-sugar-added selections are best. If you can't find canned fruits with no sugar added, eat the fruit and leave the heavy syrup behind.
- *Soups:* The sodium content can be sky high in soups, so compare labels. Pick up some prepared broth as a base for soups and to cook brown rice and other whole grains. Try simmering your whole grains in half water and half broth to boost flavor and moderate sodium. Keep a few cans of bean or lentil soup on hand to serve as part of a meal. Typically, broth-based soups are a better choice than creamy soups.
- *Nuts and nut butters:* Ideally, peanut butter, almond butter, and others should have no ingredients other than nuts and salt. All nuts are good for you, so aim for a variety. When choosing nuts, oil-roasted and dry-roasted are too similar nutritionally to make a big difference. Choose the one you prefer. Ground nut flour is nutritious and tasty in cookies and cakes, but the calories are high, so watch how much you eat. Powdered peanut butter is made from roasted peanuts that have been pressed to remove a lot of the fat before grinding into a powder. The result is a lower-fat and lower-calorie product that you can add to oatmeal, smoothies, and Asian sauces.
- *Whole grains:* There's a whole world of whole grains out there. If you haven't tried many, I encourage you to challenge

yourself every couple of weeks to pick one new whole grain or new way to eat it. Common whole grains are brown rice, wild rice, corn, popcorn, as well as products like pasta and bread that are made with whole-wheat flour. Less commonly eaten, but typically available, are quinoa, black rice, red rice, sorghum, farro, buckwheat, barley, and wheat berries. You can eat any of these in place of pasta or plain rice, add them to soups, mix them with vegetables, or use them as a foundation for a grain-based salad. To save time in meal preparation, pick up some quick-cooking or ready-to-eat whole grains. Quick-cooking whole grains may have been parboiled to reduce cooking times. Ready-to-eat whole grains are often sold in microwavable pouches and can be heated in 90 seconds or so. Double-check the sodium content to make sure it's at a reasonable level. Combinations of whole grains or whole grains and beans are also on the shelves. Again, look at the Nutrition Facts panel and ingredients list to assess the quality of the product. When it comes to pasta, whole-wheat pasta is a good choice. Like reduced-fat cheeses, they have gotten much tastier in recent years. You might want to try other whole-grain pastas, too, especially if you are intolerant to gluten. Look for pastas made from quinoa, rice, or buckwheat.

- *Bean-based pastas:* You can find pastas made of chickpeas, edamame beans, black beans, and others. Typically, they are higher in both protein and fiber than traditional pastas, but they are not usually lower in calories.
- *Cooking oils:* Liquid cooking oils are best for regular use. Canola oil has the lowest saturated fat content and the highest omega-3 fatty acid content. Olive oil has the highest amount of monounsaturated fatty acids. Extra-virgin olive oil has unique phytonutrients that may reduce inflammation. There is some controversy about extra-virgin olive oils and whether or not some products actually meet the high quality standards of extra-virgin olive oil. If you are concerned, look for a bottle

with a quality seal such as the one from the California Olive Oil Council or the International Olive Oil Council. Save walnut oil and flaxseed oil for salads and other uncooked uses. They are not stable enough for high heat.

- *Vinegars:* Pick up a couple of different types to boost flavor in your cooking and to create tasty, healthful vinaigrettes. Having at least red wine vinegar and white wine vinegar is helpful. My favorite specialty vinegar is aged balsamic. There is nothing quite like it, with its sweet taste and thick, syrupy consistency. It's perfect for drizzling over salads and fruit and for making all types of sauces. In a pinch, you can use regular balsamic vinegar by reducing it on the stove, first by bringing it to a boil and then simmering it until it's reduced in volume by half or more.

- *Condiments:* Sodium and added sugars are the likely traps here, so give the labels a careful look. Soy sauce is especially high in sodium. Choose a lower-sodium version, but compare brands first. Although it's quite high in fat, mayonnaise is made of healthful liquid oils like canola oil, so there's no need to avoid mayo. To save calories, choose a reduced-fat version and keep your portion small. Both Dijon mustard and horseradish add pizzazz to salads, vegetables, beef, chicken, and more. So does sriracha or other hot sauce. Jarred or refrigerated salsas also add interest to a variety of foods when you don't have the fresh ingredients on hand or the time to make your own. Salad dressings vary hugely in calorie content, with some as little as 50 calories per 2-tablespoon serving and others offering up three and four times that amount. If you're not up to whisking your own dressing, choose one that's lower in calories, saturated fat, sodium, and added sugars. Avoiding dressings that include cheese or bacon is a good start. There's no need to pick fat-free dressings, since some fat helps you absorb more nutrients from your other foods. Just be sure your choice is rich in healthful unsaturated fats and not the unhealthful saturated type.

- *Herbs and spices:* Herbs and spices are a necessity, starting with salt and pepper. For better taste, choose a coarse salt like kosher or sea salt. Because the flakes are larger, they have less sodium by the spoonful. These salts are not lower in sodium, however, than regular iodized salt when you measure them by weight—only when you measure them by the spoonful. Black pepper is tastier when freshly ground, so a peppermill is a good idea. But it's not always convenient when you need more than just a bit. For that reason, I buy high-quality coarse ground black pepper in a jar. If you like spice blends, read the labels carefully to pick up salt-free versions. For example, some brands of lemon pepper list salt as the second most prevalent ingredient. Surprisingly, the pricier specialty stores are often the least expensive places to buy spices. That's because you can often buy them in bulk and purchase only a spoonful or two. If you're trying out new seasonings or need just a bit for a special recipe, visit a store that sells them in bulk. Save your empty spice jars to store your bulk seasonings.
- *Beverages:* When it comes to beverages, the biggest problem for much of America is the amount of calories and added sugars in their glass. Generally, I recommend water as the go-to beverage. But, of course, other drinks have their place. Look back to the section on dairy to review options for milk and milk alternatives (page 107).
  - *Fruit juice:* Although it gets a bad reputation, 100% fruit juice usually provides the same phytonutrients present in whole fruit. Typically, the only thing lacking in juice is some or all of the dietary fiber. The problem comes when a person drinks a large amount. A small orange is the equivalent of only 1/2 cup orange juice. Too often, someone drinks a large 12-ounce glass or 20-ounce bottle of juice, which is the equivalent of three to five small oranges. For many of us, that's just too many calories in a

drink. A 4-ounce glass of fruit juice provides health-boosting phytonutrients and can fit perfectly into a balanced diet.

- *Vegetable juice:* Tomato juice and vegetable juice blends like traditional red V8 are loaded with nutrients, are low in calories, and are very filling. Compare bottles for sodium. If the low-sodium variety lacks taste, mix the low-sodium and regular varieties together or amp up the flavor with lemon juice, black pepper, horseradish, and a celery stick.
- *Sodas:* Most of America's added sugars come from sodas, energy drinks, and sports drinks. Few people other than individuals who exercise intensely benefit from sports drinks, and no one *needs* sodas or energy drinks. A 20-ounce bottle of regular soda has about 15 1/2 teaspoons of sugar! If you want a cola, ginger ale, or any other soda, it's best to have the diet version with no sugar and no calories.
- *Seltzer water:* Pick a few varieties to give you a fizzy drink without the calories and sugar. Flavors range from traditional lemon or lime to more exotic blackberry cucumber and kiwi watermelon. Double-check labels to make sure they are calorie free or nearly calorie free. You can also make your own calorie-free soda at home with a countertop soda maker.
- *Tea:* Choose tea bags or loose tea, but skip bottled teas most of the time—even the calorie-free varieties. Drinking tea is associated with diabetes prevention, reduced risks of heart attack, and perhaps even improved brain health, greater bone formation, and cancer protection. Black, green, white, and oolong teas come from the same plant and contain health-shielding phytonutrients. Drink the one you prefer, or drink a variety. Bottled teas contain little, if any, phytonutrients. Herbal teas come from other plants. Many of them have also been studied for their disease-fighting properties. Hibiscus tea, for example,

may help reduce blood pressure. Consider that some herbs interact with medications, are not recommended during pregnancy, or could have undesirable health consequences. If you have any concerns, bring them to your health care provider.

- *Coffee:* As you saw in Chapter 3, drinking coffee is linked to less risk of type 2 diabetes. In the supermarket, choose any kind of coffee you prefer other than prepared or instant coffees with added sugars or cream. Regular, decaf, plain instant, whole bean, or ground coffees are all fine. Remember to brew your coffee with a paper filter most of the time to remove the cholesterol-raising compounds.

Cooking for Health

Without a doubt, when you prepare your own meals, you have the most control over your nutrition as well as the taste of your food. To make the most of your time in the kitchen, you'll need basic cooking skills, a collection of recipes, techniques to modify less healthful recipes, and perhaps a few specialty kitchen tools.

Get Confident and Competent in the Kitchen

The best way to learn to cook or to improve your cooking skills is to cook. It's okay to feel nervous or even have a sense of dread. Just get in the kitchen and get messy. I promise that you'll find something about it that you like. For a faster and more structured path to success, check out local colleges, community centers, and cooking schools to see what cooking classes are offered in your area. Some places will have cooking classes geared to healthful eating or plant-based cooking. Others are more general. Here are a few resources to improve your kitchen skills.

Online cooking schools

- America's Test Kitchen Cooking School offers classes in basic skills such as knife skills, food safety, and how to use herbs. Other classes include the essentials of eggs, classic sauces, and comfort food makeovers. Most of their classes do not show techniques specifically for healthful cooking.
- The Roubxe online cooking school is more expensive than America's Test Kitchen Cooking School, but it offers programs in general home cooking as well as plant-based cooking.

Cookbooks

- *The Perfect Diabetes Comfort Food Collection* by Robyn Webb, MS, is not just for people with diabetes. The book starts with nine basic recipes, including lasagna, stir fry, and meatloaf, and teaches you how to make healthful variations. You'll learn tips for preparing lasagna with 10 variations, tacos with 10 variations, a burger with 10 variations, and so on.
- *Cooking Light Way to Cook* comes from the people behind *Cooking Light* magazine. Through 200+ recipes, you'll learn to steam, sauté, stir-fry, oven-fry, braise, and more. You'll also get detailed instructions on how to cut and clean leeks, slice beef into strips, seed a chile pepper, and perform many other confusing kitchen tasks.
- *Cooking Light Way to Cook Vegetarian* covers preparation techniques and recipes for eggs, tofu, tempeh, and a variety of beans and grains. Other techniques include assembling a strata, marinating tofu, and blanching vegetables.
- *How to Cook Everything* by Mark Bittman is one of the fattest cookbooks on my shelf. Its 900+ pages are filled with recipes as basic as baked potatoes and roasted chicken and as complex as Barley "Risotto" and Chicken with Indian Spices and Yogurt. Although the recipes are not specifically created with health in mind, the book is thorough with its useful descriptions of how to buy and use various types of food and perform basic cooking techniques.

Bittman covers cooking soup, vegetables, thin fish fillets, thick fish fillets, and more. It's a worthy guide despite the hefty number of recipes to avoid, such as fried chicken and hot cross buns.

- *How to Cook Everything Vegetarian* by Mark Bittman covers just about everything meatless including soups, eggs, tofu, pasta, grains, and legumes. Some recipes are too rich in saturated fat or calories (largely from cheese), but with more than 2,000 recipes and recipe variations, there's plenty to choose from. Also more than 900 pages, this book will teach you to grill and season two dozen vegetables, make fondue from chickpeas, create a variety of veggie burgers, and more.

Other publications

- *Cook's Illustrated* magazine comes out six times a year and includes detailed recipes, cooking tips, and equipment reviews. This magazine will help you develop new skills, although the recipes are not specific to healthful eating.
- *The Flavor Bible* by Karen Page and Andrew Dornenburg will help you boost your good cooking skills with new flavor profiles. There are no recipes in this book, so you are expected to already know how to cook. But use this book to up your game. Simply look up a food you want to cook and find suggestions for flavor matching from expert chefs. For example, you'll see that plums work well with arugula and prosciutto or matched with ginger and raspberries. Brussels sprouts taste great with lemon juice and thyme, and clams pair nicely with basil, garlic, and tomatoes. *The Vegetarian Flavor Bible* by Karen Page similarly matches flavors with non-meat foods.

Expand Your Recipe Repertoire

In Chapter 5, you were advised to start a healthful recipe collection. It's smart to add to the collection on a regular basis. The resources above are filled with recipes and recipe ideas, but if you just can't decide what to prepare, try to expand on your family favorites. If your family enjoys tacos, why not look for recipes for fish tacos, taco soup, and other foods along that theme? Chili fans? You should be able to find healthful recipes for chicken chili, black bean and butternut squash chili, three-bean chili, lentil chili, and so many more. In fact, later in this chapter, you'll see recipes for taco soup and lentil chili. If you have other favorite flavor combinations, look for ways to use them in different types of foods. You can borrow the ingredients of a Margherita pizza (tomatoes, basil, and mozzarella cheese) to create a salad or sandwich. Or use Greek salad staples (cucumber, onion, feta cheese, and olives) to spice up chicken or fish or to create an omelet. The possibilities are endless. If you try something new and love it, share a photo or a link on social media. Tag it with #LifestyleReset and @NutritionJill.

Strategies to "Healthify" Your Recipes and Meals

In addition to the resources above, I have several strategies to make my meals more healthful. On the following pages are 17 recipes to illustrate these strategies.

Up the Veggies

Because nonstarchy vegetables are low calorie and filling, they can help you eat a larger portion of more nutrient-dense food for fewer calories. You can trim your starch and meat servings by putting twice as much broccoli and green beans on your plate. You can try cauliflower "couscous." Plus, you can add more vegetables to existing recipes. Load up pasta and potato salads with tomatoes, broccoli, chopped red onion, and carrots. Layer thinly sliced zucchini in place of some of the noodles in your lasagna, or stuff more veggies than meat and cheese into your sandwich.

Use Lower-Fat Dairy and Meats

A simple way to cut calories and saturated fat is to remove poultry skin, select the leanest cuts of red meats, and swap full-fat dairy products for nonfat and lower-fat versions.

Cook Meats with Acids and Moist Heat

Eating huge portions of meat, even if the meat is very lean, is not smart eating. First, if we fill our plates with steak, chicken, fish, or other animal foods, it leaves less room for vegetables, beans, fruits, and whole grains—the very foods we know help prevent chronic disease. Also, meats are a main source of harmful compounds called advanced glycation end products (AGEs). These are a group of compounds present in a host of foods, but fleshy animal products are a major contributor. In small amounts, AGEs do not harm us because the body's defense mechanisms take care of them. In large amounts, however, they cause increased inflammation and insulin resistance. Not only do meats naturally contain AGEs, but AGEs are produced when meats (and cheeses) are cooked, especially with high heat and in dry conditions. You can inhibit the production of these undesirable compounds when you cook with moist heat (stewing, poaching, steaming) and when you marinate meats in acids or otherwise cook with acids like citrus juice, vinegar, tomato juice, and wine.

Eat More Legumes

Chapter 3 identifies key nutrients in beans, peas, and lentils and explains how this family of nutrient powerhouses can help prevent type 2 diabetes. If you don't eat a lot of beans now, aim for one small serving a couple times per week. Start by adding them to salads and soups and tossing them with rice and other grains. Move on to making them the center of a recipe and eating them instead of meats. In fact, I've found that lentils beautifully replace ground beef in a variety of dishes, as you'll see in the lentil chili later in this chapter.

Make Simple Substitutions

Experimenting in the kitchen will help you find more healthful and lower-calorie substitutions for common foods and ingredients. This chart also gives you a few ideas.

Simple Swaps

Instead of this . . .	Trade up with this . . .	Notes
Bottled salad dressing	Homemade vinaigrette	You control the ratio of oil to vinegar or lemon juice
Mayonnaise	Reduced-fat mayonnaise	Fewer calories
		Try different brands to find one you like
Sour cream	Reduced-fat or fat-free sour cream	Fewer calories and less saturated fat
		Avoid fat-free sour cream in savory recipes because it may sweeten your dish
	Reduced-fat or fat-free strained (Greek or Icelandic) yogurt	Fewer calories and less saturated fat; more protein
Sugar in baking	Reduce the sugar by 1/4 to 1/3 or cut sugar in half and use a combination of sugar and sugar substitute	Sweetness can be intensified with the addition of cinnamon, nutmeg, or vanilla extract or by sprinkling a small amount of sugar on top just before or after baking

(Continued on next page)

Instead of this . . .	Trade up with this . . .	Notes
Breadcrumbs	Rolled oats or crushed bran cereal	Less refined flour; more vitamins, minerals, fiber, and phytonutrients
	Chopped walnuts or other nuts	Less refined flour; more healthy fats, vitamins, minerals, fiber, and phytonutrients
White flour	White whole-wheat flour	More vitamins, minerals, fiber
	Whole-wheat flour or whole-wheat pastry flour	More vitamins, minerals, fiber, and phytonutrients
Butter or shortening in baking	Replace 4 tablespoons hard fat with 3 tablespoons canola oil	Less saturated fat; more healthy fats
	Replace hard fat with an equal amount of mashed avocado	Less saturated fat; more healthy fats, vitamins, minerals, fiber, and phytonutrients
Butter in cooking	Olive, canola, or other cooking oils (not coconut oil)	Less saturated fat; more healthy fats
Butter on toast	Any nut butter, peanut butter, or sunflower butter	Less saturated fat; more healthy fats, protein, vitamins, minerals, fiber, and phytonutrients

Instead of this . . .	Trade up with this . . .	Notes
	Mashed avocado	Less saturated fat; more healthy fats, vitamins, minerals, fiber, and phytonutrients
		Get creative with the addition of other vegetables and fresh herbs on top of the avocado
Cheddar cheese in recipes, 1 oz	3/4 oz sharp cheddar cheese	The sharp cheese has a stronger flavor, so you can use less
Cheese on sandwiches	Reduced-fat cheese	Less saturated fat and fewer calories
	Avocado	Less saturated fat; more healthy fats, fiber, and phytonutrients and a different array of vitamins and minerals
Cream in soups and sauces	Milk or nonfat plain Greek yogurt	Less saturated fat; more protein
	Alternatively, thicken soups with pureed vegetables or smashed beans	Less saturated fat; more fiber, vitamins, minerals, and phytonutrients

(Continued on next page)

Instead of this . . .	Trade up with this . . .	Notes
Cream sauce (like Alfredo) on pasta	Tomato-based sauce	Less saturated fat and fewer calories; more vitamins, minerals, fiber, and phytonutrients
	Olive oil and garlic	Less saturated fat; more healthy fats, and phytonutrients
		Olive oil is calorie-dense, so watch the total amount
Oil in marinades	Decrease oil by 1/4 to 1/2	Flavored vinegars, citrus juices, and wine also make good marinades
Oil in pan cooking	Sauté in half the oil. Deglaze the pan with broth or wine if the food sticks.	Using a good-quality nonstick pan helps when decreasing the oil
Poultry with the skin	Poultry without the skin	To keep the meat moist, remove the skin before eating, use seasoned crumbs on skinless poultry before cooking, or cook with moist heat
Prime rib	Eye of round	Generally, any cut of beef with "loin" or "round" is a lean cut

Instead of this . . .	Trade up with this . . .	Notes
Regular ground beef	Ground meat at least 90% lean	Read labels for ground turkey
		Some are high in calories and fat because it is ground with the skin
	You can also extend your ground beef with lentils, beans, diced mushrooms, shredded zucchini, or other vegetable	Less saturated fat and fewer calories; more vitamins, minerals, fiber, and phytonutrients
Soups and stews	Prepare soups and stews a day early	Fat rises to the top and hardens, making it easy to skim the fat
Onion dip	Hummus	Less saturated fat; more healthy fats, protein, fiber, and phytonutrients
Cheese dip	Guacamole	Less saturated fat and fewer calories; more healthy fats, vitamins, minerals, fiber, and phytonutrients
Fruit-on-the-bottom yogurt	Nonfat or low-fat strained yogurt (Greek or Icelandic) and fresh fruit	Fewer calories and less added sugar; more vitamins, minerals, fiber, and phytonutrients
Large bagel	English muffin, small bagel, or bagel thins	Cuts calories by about half; best to choose whole-grain options

(Continued on next page)

Instead of this . . .	Trade up with this . . .	Notes
Snack crackers	Whole-grain crackers	No refined grains; more vitamins, minerals, fiber, and phytonutrients
	Almonds, pistachios, peanuts, walnuts, or other nuts or roasted chickpeas	No refined grains; more healthy fats, vitamins, minerals, fiber, and phytonutrients
		Eat them in preportioned packages to keep calories in check
Instant flavored oatmeal	Instant plain oatmeal	Fewer calories and less added sugar
	1-minute oats	Fewer calories and less added sugar and sodium
White rice	Brown rice, wild rice, barley, quinoa, farro, freekeh	No refined grains; more vitamins, minerals, fiber, and phytonutrients
		Cook these in half water and half broth to add flavor with minimum sodium
	Cauliflower "couscous"	Fewer calories; more vitamins, minerals, fiber, and phytonutrients

Kitchen Tools Worth the Space

Cooking is easier and more fun when you have the right tools. The appliances and utensils you'll need depend so much on the types of foods you prepare and your style of cooking. There's no ideal list of tools, but below are several that are typically useful. Give careful thought to how you'll use each item before you decide if it's worth the expense and space.

Rice Cooker

A rice cooker is an ideal appliance to cook any number of grains including oats, quinoa, wheat berries, farro, freekeh, and, of course, rice. It frees up your stove for other cooking, and it turns itself off when your grain is ready to eat.

Slow Cooker or Crock-Pot

Slow cookers are handy for stews, soups, beef roasts, and even casseroles and side dishes. As long as you plan ahead, you can come home at the end of the day to delicious smells and ready-to-eat food.

Multi-Cooker or Pressure Cooker

These handy appliances cook food quickly. An multi-cooker typically functions as a pressure cooker, slow cooker, and a rice cooker. A pressure cooker has just the one function.

Immersion Blender

Immersion blenders are also known as stick blenders and are very handy for a quick smoothie. These devices let you blend right in the pot for a pureed soup or vegetable.

Industrial-Strength Blender

This pricey piece of equipment is a huge workhorse in the kitchen, especially if you use a lot of whole foods and cook mostly from scratch.

It turns nuts into nut butters, vegetables into soups, beans into purees for veggie burgers, and chicken and vegetables into chicken salad lickety-split. These blenders make beautiful smoothies, too.

Food Processor

Use a food processor to quickly slice, dice, and shred food. If space is tight, consider purchasing a mini–food processor.

Panini Press

You'll turn an everyday sandwich into something delicious and nutritious when you slip some reduced-fat cheese along with fruits or vegetables and fresh herbs between two slices of whole-grain bread and press it until warm and toasty.

Hand Juicer

Trim salt and make flavors pop with a squeeze of fresh lemon or other citrus. Try citrus juice in soups and stews and over vegetables, whole grains, meats, and more.

Other Favorite Kitchen Tools

Here are other tools that you'll likely use on a regular basis: measuring cups and spoons, digital food scale, heat-resistant spatulas and spoons, tongs, nonstick baking mat, a salad spinner, colanders, digital timer, digital thermometer, cutting boards, kitchen shears, vegetable peeler, and a vegetable steamer.

Recipes

You'll find 17 recipes below to serve as inspiration in your own cooking. In each recipe, I point out the changes I made to make the dish more wholesome than a traditional version. Sometimes the calories, saturated fat, or sodium is reduced. Sometimes health-shielding ingre-dients are added. And some recipes involve a combination of tech-niques, but none is truly unique. I include them and point them out, so you can get ideas to tweak your own favorite recipes. You will see these same strategies to "healthify" recipes in plenty of cookbooks and magazines. If something seems a bit strange, keep an open mind and try it when you know there will be plenty of other foods to enjoy. That way, if you end up not liking a recipe or a strategy to healthify, you and your family won't go hungry. Chances are, though, you'll find a new way to boost nutrition that you can use every time you cook.

At the end of the chapter, I've included some sample menus, also to serve as inspiration when meal planning.

Cheers to happy, healthful eating!

Enjoy the following recipes:

Veggie-Packed Potato Salad
Chunky Gazpacho
Veggie-Heavy Spaghetti Sauce
Citrus and Herb Chicken Thighs
Turkey Taco Soup
Cauliflower Couscous
Lentil and Sweet Potato Chili
Lemon Basil Sauce for Fish
Southwestern Macaroni and Cheese
Roasted Vegetables
Mason Jar Salad
Nourish Meal Bowl
Avocado Cream Dressing or Sauce
Greek Salad Dressing
Mixed Berry Frozen Yogurt
Chocolate Walnut Date Balls
Apricot-Cherry Almond Balls

Veggie-Packed Potato Salad

YIELD: about 7 cups

SERVES: 6   SERVING SIZE: about 1 1/8 cups

PREP TIME: 20 minutes   COOKING TIME: 11 minutes

This recipe originally appeared in *Diabetes Weight Loss: Week by Week*. Eating this dish is a nice way to enjoy potatoes because cooked and cooled potatoes offer a bit of health-boosting resistant starch. For such a hefty portion, it serves up relatively few calories. Each bite is packed with potatoes as well as other vegetables, giving you more volume and nutrition for fewer calories. And I used an oil and vinegar dressing instead of mayonnaise to get more coverage for less fat and calories. Feel free to mix up the vegetables. Try blanched asparagus and halved cherry tomatoes. Once you see how easy it is to bulk up your favorite recipes with nonstarchy vegetables, you can use this trick with any number of family favorites.

INGREDIENTS

1 1/2 pounds red-skinned potatoes, cut in large bite-sized pieces
4 ounces snow peas, trimmed and cut in bite-sized pieces (about 1 1/4 cups)
3 tablespoons olive oil
3 tablespoons seasoned rice vinegar
1/2 teaspoon kosher salt
1/8–1/4 teaspoon black pepper
1 teaspoon Dijon mustard
4 scallions, chopped (about 1/2 cup)
1 cup chopped red or orange bell pepper
1/2 cup chopped parsley

INSTRUCTIONS

1. Place the potatoes in a large saucepan and cover with water. Bring to a boil, and then reduce heat so the water bubbles gently. Cook until potatoes are nearly at desired tenderness, about 10 minutes, but you will have to test them frequently to avoid overcooking. Just before the potatoes are done, drop the snow peas in the pot and cook for 30–60 seconds until they are slightly softer, but sill crunchy. Drain and rinse in cold water to stop the cooking process.

2. While the potatoes are cooking, whisk the oil, vinegar, salt, black pepper, and mustard together.

3. Once the potatoes and snow peas are well drained, put them in a large bowl with the scallions, bell pepper, and parsley. Pour the dressing over the potatoes and vegetables and mix gently. Chill well before serving.

CHOICES
1 1/2 Starch, 1 Nonstarchy Vegetable, 1 Fat

BASIC NUTRITIONAL VALUES

Calories	180	**Potassium**	570 mg
Calories from Fat	60	**Total Carbohydrate**	26 g
Total Fat	7.0 g	Dietary Fiber	4 g
Saturated Fat	1.0 g	Sugars	3 g
Trans Fat	0.0 g	**Protein**	3 g
Cholesterol	0 mg	**Phosphorus**	75 mg
Sodium	190 mg		

Chunky Gazpacho

YIELD: about 9 cups

SERVES: 9

SERVING SIZE: about 1 1/8 cups

PREP TIME: 15 minutes plus chilling time

COOKING TIME: None

It's all vegetables here! My family adores this recipe, so I make it three or four times a month in the summer. I have a Vitamix, so it comes together super fast. We enjoy this recipe for lunch and dinner and as a cool, filling, hydrating snack. If you prefer a smoother gazpacho, keep processing until you get just the consistency you want. For a creamier texture, you can add a slice of bread shortly before processing. If you want to trim the sodium even more, use a lower-sodium vegetable juice or mix the lower-sodium and regular varieties together.

INGREDIENTS

1 1/2 pounds ripe tomatoes

1 medium cucumber

1 large sweet onion, peeled

1 1/2 large bell peppers, any color

2 large celery stalks

2 garlic cloves

2 tablespoons extra-virgin olive oil

1 tablespoon balsamic vinegar

1 tablespoon rice vinegar

4–6 fresh basil leaves

1/2 teaspoon sriracha or hot pepper sauce, to taste

1/2 teaspoon ground black pepper

22 fluid ounces vegetable juice, such as V8 Original Vegetable Juice, divided

INSTRUCTIONS

1 Cut the vegetables into manageable pieces, usually about 2 or 3 inches each.

2 Place all of the ingredients except the vegetable or tomato juice in a high-powered blender like a Vitamix or a food processor. Add about half of the vegetable juice. Process until you have very small pieces and the desired consistency.

3 Add the rest of the vegetable juice. Stir. Taste and adjust seasonings if necessary. Refrigerate a few hours until it is very cold.

4 Serve as is or add diced avocado, red onion, and snipped basil.

CHOICES
2 Nonstarchy Vegetable, 1/2 Fat

BASIC NUTRITIONAL VALUES

Calories	90	**Potassium**	510 mg
Calories from Fat	30	**Total Carbohydrate**	13 g
Total Fat	3.5 g	Dietary Fiber	3 g
Saturated Fat	0.5 g	Sugars	8 g
Trans Fat	0.0 g	**Protein**	2 g
Cholesterol	0 mg	**Phosphorus**	60 mg
Sodium	220 mg		

Veggie-Heavy Spaghetti Sauce

YIELD: 7 cups

SERVES: 6   SERVING SIZE: 1 rounded cup

PREP TIME: 12 minutes   COOKING TIME: 20 minutes

This is leaner and has fewer calories than traditional meat sauce because of my choice of 93% lean beef. But the addition of the vegetables really makes this recipe unique, giving you a bigger portion for fewer calories and greater nutrition. Feel free to add any favorite vegetable and in any quantity that makes sense to you. For this version, I've chosen zucchini and carrots to equal about 2 1/2–3 cups uncooked vegetables.

INGREDIENTS

1 pound 93% lean ground beef

1 small yellow onion, chopped (1 scant cup)

2 garlic cloves, crushed or chopped

1 (24-ounce) bottle reduced-sodium pasta sauce, such as marinara or tomato basil

1 (14.5-ounce) can petite diced no-salt-added tomatoes, undrained

1 large carrot, chopped

2 large zucchini, cut in half lengthwise, then cut into 1/2-inch slices

INSTRUCTIONS

1 Add the meat to a large skillet on medium-high heat, and break up the meat quickly. Add the onion and cook until the meat is browned, about 4 minutes. Add the garlic and stir.

2 Add the jarred pasta sauce and the canned tomatoes. Stir. Increase the heat to high.

3 Add the carrots or any firm vegetable you choose to use. Stir and cook about 1–2 minutes. Add the zucchini or other softer vegetable. Stir. Reduce the heat to a simmer. Cover and cook, stirring periodically, about 10–12 minutes until the sauce is thick and the vegetables are tender.

CHOICES
1/2 Starch, 2 Nonstarchy Vegetable, 2 Protein, lean, 1 Fat

BASIC NUTRITIONAL VALUES

Calories	230	**Potassium**	1060 mg
Calories from Fat	90	**Total Carbohydrate**	18 g
Total Fat	10.0 g	Dietary Fiber	4 g
Saturated Fat	2.7 g	Sugars	11 g
Trans Fat	0.3 g	**Protein**	19 g
Cholesterol	45 mg	**Phosphorus**	230 mg
Sodium	370 mg		

Citrus and Herb Chicken Thighs

YIELD: 18 ounces of chicken, 12 tablespoons sauce

SERVES: 6

SERVING SIZE: about 3 ounces of chicken and 2 tablespoons sauce

PREP TIME: 10 minutes plus chilling time

COOKING TIME: 30 minutes

Earlier in this chapter, we discussed a group of harmful compounds called advanced glycation end products, or AGEs for short. Meats are a main source of AGEs, and this is likely one reason that plant-based diets are linked to less chronic disease. We can stop additional AGEs from forming by cooking with moist heat and acids. This recipe uses both.

INGREDIENTS

1 1/2 pounds boneless, skinless chicken thighs

1/4 teaspoon kosher salt

1/4 teaspoon coarse ground black pepper

1/2 cup orange juice

4 cloves garlic, crushed or chopped

1 tablespoon Italian seasonings

1 teaspoon dried rosemary

1 teaspoon dried thyme

1/4 teaspoon red pepper flakes

1 tablespoon brown sugar

1 small yellow onion, chopped (scant 1 cup)

2 medium oranges, sliced

2 medium lemons, sliced

INSTRUCTIONS

1 Place the chicken thighs single layer in a 9 × 13-inch baking pan. Sprinkle with salt and pepper.

2 In a medium bowl, whisk together the next 7 ingredients (orange juice through brown sugar). Add the chopped onion. Pour the mixture evenly over the chicken.

3 Cover the chicken with the orange and lemon slices. If you have time, refrigerate for 1 hour or overnight. Bake at 375°F for 25–30 minutes until the chicken is tender and cooked through.

CHOICES
1/2 Fruit, 1/2 Carbohydrate, 3 Protein, lean

BASIC NUTRITIONAL VALUES

Calories	190	**Potassium**	400 mg
Calories from Fat	60	**Total Carbohydrate**	14 g
Total Fat	7.0 g	Dietary Fiber	2 g
Saturated Fat	1.8 g	Sugars	9 g
Trans Fat	0.0 g	**Protein**	19 g
Cholesterol	105 mg	**Phosphorus**	185 mg
Sodium	150 mg		

Turkey Taco Soup

YIELD: 10 1/2 cups

SERVES: 7   SERVING SIZE: 1 1/2 cups

PREP TIME: 12 minutes   COOKING TIME: 38 minutes

This is a great way for meat lovers to get some health-boosting beans. I've made the soup a bit brothy to keep the calories low and the portions large and filling. By using both broth and water, I'm able to serve up a large portion while keeping the sodium levels moderate.

INGREDIENTS

1 pound 93% lean ground turkey

1 medium yellow onion, chopped (about 1 1/2 cups)

1 large green bell pepper, chopped (about 1 cup)

4 garlic cloves, crushed or chopped

1 tablespoon chili powder

1 teaspoon ground cumin

1/2 teaspoon dried oregano

1/4 teaspoon cayenne pepper

1 (15.5-ounce) can no-salt-added red kidney beans, drained and rinsed

1 (14.5-ounce) can petite diced no-salt-added tomatoes, undrained

5 cups reduced-sodium chicken broth

1 cup water

1/2 cup nonfat plain Greek yogurt

1/4 cup cilantro, chopped

INSTRUCTIONS

1 In a large pot over medium-high heat, brown the meat and soften the onions and bell pepper, about 7 minutes.

2 Add the garlic, chili powder, cumin, oregano, and cayenne pepper. Stir. Add the beans, tomatoes, broth, and water. Stir.

3 Cover and bring to a boil. Reduce the heat and simmer about 30 minutes.

4 Garnish each serving as desired with 1 tablespoon nonfat Greek yogurt, chopped cilantro, etc.

CHOICES
1/2 Starch, 2 Nonstarchy Vegetable, 2 Protein, lean, 1/2 Fat

BASIC NUTRITIONAL VALUES

Calories	210	**Potassium**	720 mg
Calories from Fat	45	**Total Carbohydrate**	18 g
Total Fat	5.0 g	Dietary Fiber	5 g
Saturated Fat	1.5 g	Sugars	6 g
Trans Fat	0.1 g	**Protein**	21 g
Cholesterol	50 mg	**Phosphorus**	265 mg
Sodium	500 mg		

Cauliflower Couscous

YIELD: 3 cups

SERVES: 4   SERVING SIZE: 3/4 cup

PREP TIME: 5 minutes   COOKING TIME: 13 minutes

Many people call this cauliflower rice, but the texture is much more like couscous than rice. Once you get the basic recipe down, you'll find many variations to enjoy. For example, change up the spices to match the other foods in your meal. When I make chicken with paprika, I serve it over cauliflower couscous seasoned with garlic, paprika, and cayenne pepper. But if I were going to serve it with crab cakes, I might season the cauliflower couscous with dill and lemon zest.

Ingredient note: You can usually find "riced" cauliflower in the produce section of your grocery store. Alternatively, you can rice your own cauliflower. Simply wash a head of cauliflower and cut it into 4 to 6 chunks. Using a food processor with a mixing blade, process the cauliflower until the pieces are the size of rice.

INGREDIENTS

1 tablespoon canola or extra-virgin olive oil

1 small yellow onion, chopped (1 scant cup)

1 pound "riced" cauliflower (about 4 cups)

2 garlic cloves, crushed or chopped

1/2 teaspoon dried thyme

1/2 teaspoon coarse ground black pepper

1/4 teaspoon kosher salt

INSTRUCTIONS

1 Heat a medium nonstick skillet over medium heat. Add the oil and swirl to cover the pan. Sauté the onion until soft, about 5 minutes. Add the garlic and stir. Add the cauliflower and the spices. Stir.

2 Turn the heat to medium high and cook until the cauliflower is soft and slightly browned, about 5–7 minutes.

CHOICES
2 Nonstarchy Vegetable, 1 Fat

BASIC NUTRITIONAL VALUES

Calories	80	**Potassium**	450 mg
Calories from Fat	35	**Total Carbohydrate**	10 g
Total Fat	4.0 g	Dietary Fiber	3 g
Saturated Fat	0.4 g	Sugars	4 g
Trans Fat	0.0 g	**Protein**	3 g
Cholesterol	0 mg	**Phosphorus**	70 mg
Sodium	160 mg		

Lentil and Sweet Potato Chili

YIELD: 10–11 cups
SERVES: 7   SERVING SIZE: 1 1/2 cups
PREP TIME: 18 minutes   COOKING TIME: 57 minutes

I continue to be surprised by how well lentils substitute for ground beef or ground turkey in a host of recipes. I've made lentil sloppy joes and lentil spaghetti sauce, and I use lentils in a bunch of other ways, too. It's really not that hard to adapt other recipe concepts to use these health-boosting, disease-fighting legumes. Give it a try. In this recipe, as in others, I've combined lower-sodium and regular products to bring the total sodium down. This is a great way to gradually lower the sodium in your typical recipes and help family members adjust to the change in taste. Use the combination that works for you and those you cook for with the idea that, bit by bit, you can trim sodium to an appropriate level. This recipe makes a very big pot. I adore the cook-once, eat-often strategy! My husband and I both really enjoy having this chili leftover for lunch. If you're not a leftovers fan, simply cut the recipe in half or freeze what's left over. In a pinch, you can omit the tomato paste, but I think it adds a wonderful meaty taste to this vegetarian dish. Top the chili with your favorite chili toppings such as diced avocado, scallions, cilantro, and nonfat Greek yogurt. I especially like the yogurt to boost the protein content.

INGREDIENTS

1 tablespoon canola or extra-virgin olive oil
1 very large onion, chopped (about 2 1/2 cups)
3 large carrots chopped (about 1 cup)
2 large bell peppers, cut into bite-sized pieces (about 2 cups)
4 garlic cloves, chopped or crushed
2 tablespoons tomato paste
1 large sweet potato (about 16 ounces), peeled and cut into bite-sized
    pieces (about 3 cups)

1 tablespoon chili powder

1 1/4 teaspoon ground cumin

1 teaspoon dried oregano

1/4 teaspoon cayenne pepper

1 cup green lentils, dry

1 (14.5-ounce) can petite diced tomatoes, undrained

12 fluid ounces low-sodium vegetable juice

2 cups regular vegetable broth

2 cups low-sodium vegetable broth

INSTRUCTIONS

1　Heat the oil in a Dutch oven or a large pot with a lid over medium heat. Sauté the onions, carrots, and bell peppers until soft, about 7–8 minutes. Add the garlic and the tomato paste. Stir about 30 seconds.

2　Add the sweet potato and the spices (chili powder through cayenne pepper). Stir. Add the lentils, tomatoes, vegetable juice, and both types of vegetable broth. Raise the heat to a boil. Reduce the heat to a low boil. Cover and cook for about 45 minutes or until the chili is thick and the lentils are soft.

CHOICES
2 Starch, 3 Nonstarchy Vegetable

BASIC NUTRITIONAL VALUES

Calories	230	**Potassium**	1050 mg
Calories from Fat	25	**Total Carbohydrate**	43 g
Total Fat	3.0 g	Dietary Fiber	12 g
Saturated Fat	0.3 g	Sugars	14 g
Trans Fat	0.0 g	**Protein**	10 g
Cholesterol	0 mg	**Phosphorus**	250 mg
Sodium	463 mg		

Lemon Basil Sauce for Fish

YIELD: 5 tablespoons

SERVES: 4   SERVING SIZE: 3 3/4 teaspoons

PREP TIME: 5 minutes   COOKING TIME: None

Adding this sauce is one of my favorite ways to eat salmon, although it's tasty with a variety of fish. The presentation of the dish is pretty, too, so it's perfect for company. Before baking or grilling your fish, squeeze a lemon over it. When finished cooking, pour this sauce over the fish and serve. Be sure to use a good-quality olive oil.

INGREDIENTS

3 tablespoons lemon juice

2 tablespoons extra-virgin olive oil

4 garlic cloves, crushed or chopped

1/8 cup packed chopped fresh basil leaves

INSTRUCTIONS

1 Whisk all of the ingredients together. Pour over prepared fish just before serving.

CHOICES
1 1/2 Fat

BASIC NUTRITIONAL VALUES

Calories	70	**Potassium**	35 mg
Calories from Fat	60	**Total Carbohydrate**	2 g
Total Fat	7.0 g	Dietary Fiber	0 g
Saturated Fat	0.9 g	Sugars	0 g
Trans Fat	0.0 g	**Protein**	0 g
Cholesterol	0 mg	**Phosphorus**	5 mg
Sodium	0 mg		

Southwestern Macaroni and Cheese

YIELD: 8 cups
SERVES: 16   SERVING SIZE: 1/2 cup
PREP TIME: 5 minutes   COOKING TIME: 54 minutes

This recipe is hugely trimmed of saturated fat, but is still creamy and flavorful and a good addition to your next potluck. Nonfat milk and reduced-fat cheese make it happen. Using whole-grain pasta boosts the fiber, and the spices and vegetables make it interesting. Use this recipe as a template for a host of variations. Skip the southwestern flavors in favor of other tastes, depending on your mood. I've made a similar dish with a Mediterranean flair to include spinach, tomatoes, kalamata olives, and feta cheese.

INGREDIENTS

8 ounces dry whole-grain pasta shells or elbow macaroni
1/4 cup all-purpose flour
1 3/4 cups nonfat milk
10 ounces reduced-fat sharp cheddar cheese, shredded (2 1/2 cups)
3 garlic cloves, crushed or chopped
1/2 teaspoon coarse black pepper
1 teaspoon chili powder
1 (14.5-ounce) can petite diced no-salt-added tomatoes, drained
1 (4-ounce) can diced green chile peppers

INSTRUCTIONS

1 Preheat the oven to 375°F. Cook the pasta according to package directions, but without salt or fat. Drain and set aside.

2 Place the flour in a large pot over medium heat. Gradually add the milk and whisk briskly. Stir until thickened, about 4–6 minutes. Remove the pot from the heat.

3 Add the cheese and stir until melted and evenly dispersed. Add the garlic, black pepper, and chili powder. Stir. Add the tomatoes and chile peppers. Mix thoroughly.

4 Pour the contents into a 2.5-liter (about 10 cups) casserole dish that has been prepared with nonstick pan spray. Bake uncovered for 35 minutes.

CHOICES
1 Starch, 1 Protein, lean

BASIC NUTRITIONAL VALUES

Calories	120	**Potassium**	170 mg
Calories from Fat	40	**Total Carbohydrate**	14 g
Total Fat	4.5 g	Dietary Fiber	2.1 g
Saturated Fat	2.3 g	Sugars	2 g
Trans Fat	0.0 g	**Protein**	8 g
Cholesterol	10 mg	**Phosphorus**	185 mg
Sodium	190 mg		

Roasted Vegetables

This is not a recipe per se. Rather, it's general instructions to roast a variety of vegetables. Roasted vegetables are easy to prepare, and they can make most anyone a fan of vegetables. Roasting brings out a vegetable's natural sweet taste.

INSTRUCTIONS

1 Preheat the oven to 425°F. Cut the vegetables into uniform pieces. I prefer mine on the large size, so I might cut broccoli into 3-inch pieces and leave asparagus whole.

2 Dry the vegetables thoroughly. Then toss with olive oil and seasonings of your choice. Some examples for inspiration:

- Broccoli with salt and red pepper flakes
- Cauliflower with salt and thyme
- Green beans with salt and tarragon
- Butternut squash with sage or coriander

3 Spread the vegetables onto a baking sheet or two. Do not crowd the pan or the vegetables will steam instead of roast, and you'll be left without the caramelized goodness. Roast until brown and tender, turning once or twice. The amount of time it takes to cook your vegetables will depend on the type of vegetable and the size of the pieces. I typically cook large pieces of broccoli and cauliflower for a total of 20–25 minutes, turning after about 15 minutes. Smaller and softer vegetables might be done in as little as 10 minutes. Check your vegetables and move them around on the pan after about 10 minutes. Continue until browned and tender.

4 Often, a squeeze of fresh lemon just before serving brightens the flavors even more, especially on green vegetables.

Mason Jar Salad

This too is just a set of general instructions to help you layer your ingredients in just the right order to keep your salad fresh, not limp. Get creative to prepare any kind of salad you like. Make a few on Sunday to have for work for the next several days.

INSTRUCTIONS

1   Start with a clean, dry mason jar with a lid. Then add ingredients in the following order. Feel free to omit anything you don't want in your salad.

- A tablespoon or two of salad dressing
- Hard vegetables and fruits such as carrots, celery, cabbage, apple, and the like
- Black beans, chickpeas, and other beans
- Cooked grains like farro, quinoa, pasta, or rice
- Softer vegetables and fruits such as tomatoes, avocado, strawberries, blueberries, and peaches
- Meats, cheeses, and hard-boiled egg

2   Fill to the top with leafy greens such as arugula, spinach, or lettuce.

3   If you won't be eating your salad within a day or two, omit the meats and egg. Add them on top of the leafy greens in the morning of the day you plan to eat your salad.

4   Before eating, shake the salad and pour it onto a plate or bowl. Use a fork to mix the salad.

Nourish Meal Bowl

Here's one more recipe blueprint. These instructions guide you in creating a nourishing, tasty meal in the convenience of a single bowl. I love this idea as a way to use leftovers, but the bowl is also a terrific way to exercise your creativity. Your bowl can take on the flavors of any country or region that interests you, or it can simply be a combination of favorite foods or even just a method of cleaning out your refrigerator. In fact, the nourish meal bowl concept is so versatile that you can have each member of the family create a unique masterpiece. The point is that you include all key components of a meal: lots of vegetables, a starchy food, and a protein-rich food. If desired, you can further round out your meal with a piece of fruit and a glass of milk.

INSTRUCTIONS

Add the following types of ingredients in the amounts suitable to your preferences and needs. If you're using both hot and cold ingredients, heat the hot ingredients separately before putting them in the bowl. You can layer each ingredient, mix all of them together, or place each ingredient side by side, which I think makes a prettier bowl.

- A whole grain or starchy vegetable such as brown rice, quinoa, farro, or roasted sweet potatoes
- Cooked or raw leafy greens (or both) such as kale, spinach, arugula, or Swiss chard
- Additional cooked vegetable such as roasted Brussels sprouts, carrots, or broccoli, or sautéed onions and bell pepper
- A protein-rich food such as baked salmon, rotisserie chicken, canned tuna, roasted tofu, lentils, or black beans
- A source of healthy fats such as avocado, nuts, or seeds
- Extras: Make this a meal to look forward to by including favorites such as dried fruit, fresh fruit, additional raw vegetables, sauerkraut, hummus, or fresh herbs.

- Dressing or sauce such as bottled ginger dressing, packaged tzatziki, fruit or vegetable salsa, creamy avocado dressing, spicy peanut sauce, or pesto sauce

Here are some combinations just to get you started. You should use the ingredients that are convenient for you.

1. Farro, spinach, sautéed onions and bell peppers, leftover chicken, corn, black beans, avocado, salsa
2. Quinoa, arugula, roasted broccoli, roasted tofu, peanuts, peanut sauce
3. Brown rice, kale, roasted butternut squash and mushrooms, chickpeas, tahini dressing
4. Leftover pasta, sautéed spinach, leftover salmon, cannellini beans, toasted walnuts, berries, feta cheese, fresh basil, drizzle of extra-virgin olive oil and lemon juice

Avocado Cream Dressing or Sauce

YIELD: 10 Tablespoons

SERVES: 5   SERVING SIZE: 2 Tablespoons

PREP TIME: 8 minutes   COOKING TIME: None

This quick-to-prepare whole foods sauce is perfect to dress a salad or top a piece of baked fish. It even works well mixed into riced cauliflower.

INGREDIENTS ———————————————————————————————

1 medium avocado, peeled and pitted

1/4 cup nonfat, plain strained yogurt (Greek or Icelandic)

1/2 cup packed fresh cilantro or basil

Juice of 1/2 lime (about 1 tablespoon)

1 garlic clove

INSTRUCTIONS

1 Place all of the ingredients in a food processor.

2 Pulse on and off until you have a smooth consistency.

CHOICES
1 Fat

BASIC NUTRITIONAL VALUES

Calories	60		**Potassium**	200 mg
Calories from Fat	40		**Total Carbohydrate**	4 g
Total Fat	4.5 g		Dietary Fiber	2 g
Saturated Fat	0.7 g		Sugars	1 g
Trans Fat	0.0 g		**Protein**	2 g
Cholesterol	0 mg		**Phosphorus**	35 mg
Sodium	10 mg			

Greek Salad Dressing

YIELD: 12 Tablespoons

SERVES: 8   **SERVING SIZE:** 1 1/2 Tablespoons

PREP TIME: 6 minutes   **COOKING TIME:** None

Use this dressing in a Greek Mason Jar Salad (see page 155) or mix up the spices to suit another flavor profile. Instead of some or all of the lemon juice, you might like red wine vinegar.

INGREDIENTS

2 garlic cloves, crushed or chopped

1 teaspoon dried oregano

1/2 teaspoon Dijon mustard

1/2 teaspoon kosher salt

1/2 teaspoon coarse black pepper

4 tablespoons lemon juice

8 tablespoons extra-virgin olive oil

INSTRUCTIONS

1 Whisk together all of the ingredients except the olive oil.

2 While continuing to whisk, slowly pour in the olive oil.

3 Refrigerate the leftovers.

CHOICES
3 Fat

BASIC NUTRITIONAL VALUES

Calories	120	**Potassium**	15 mg
Calories from Fat	130	**Total Carbohydrate**	1 g
Total Fat	14.0 g	Dietary Fiber	0 g
Saturated Fat	1.9 g	Sugars	0 g
Trans Fat	0.0 g	**Protein**	0 g
Cholesterol	0 mg	**Phosphorus**	5 mg
Sodium	130 mg		

Mixed Berry Frozen Yogurt

YIELD: 1 cup

SERVES: 2

PREP TIME: 5 minutes

SERVING SIZE: 1/2 cup

FREEZING TIME: At least 2 hours

I'm a big fan of desserts with benefits. And I have several that I truly love, including homemade frozen yogurt. Treat yourself to something sweet with the knowledge that you're also eating wholesome foods.

INGREDIENTS

1 cup frozen mixed berries or mixed berries with cherries (about 4.7 ounces)

1 (5.3-ounce) container of nonfat strawberry Greek or Icelandic yogurt

INSTRUCTIONS

1   Place both ingredients into a food processor or powerful blender and mix thoroughly.

2   Transfer the contents into a freezer-safe container, and freeze for at least 2 hours.

3   If desired, garnish with fresh mint leaves or chocolate shavings.

CHOICES
1/2 Fruit, 1/2 Milk, fat-free

BASIC NUTRITIONAL VALUES

Calories	90	Potassium	200 mg
Calories from Fat	0	Total Carbohydrate	15 g
Total Fat	0.0 g	Dietary Fiber	3 g
Saturated Fat	0.1 g	Sugars	10 g
Trans Fat	0.0 g	Protein	8 g
Cholesterol	0 mg	Phosphorus	120 mg
Sodium	25 mg		

Chocolate Walnut Date Balls

YIELD: 18 balls

SERVES: 9　　　　SERVING SIZE: 2 balls

PREP TIME: 15 minutes　　COOKING TIME: None

This little dessert with benefits is loaded with health-shielding nutrients and a delicious chocolate taste.

INGREDIENTS ————————————————————————

1 cup pitted sticky dates such as Medjool or Deglet Noor (4.5 ounces)

1/2 cup raisins (2.3 ounces)

1/2 cup walnuts (2 ounces)

2 tablespoons cocoa powder

1/4 cup chocolate chips (1.5 ounces)

1 tablespoon water

INSTRUCTIONS

1 Using a food processor, process everything except the water until finely chopped.

2 Add the water and process again for several seconds until you have a sticky mass.

3 Using damp hands, form 18 (1-inch) balls, each weighing about 18 grams.

4 Place the balls in a container with a lid. Separate layers with wax paper. Store at room temperature or the refrigerator.

CHOICES
1 Fruit, 1/2 Carbohydrate, 1 Fat

BASIC NUTRITIONAL VALUES

Calories	130	**Potassium**	210 mg
Calories from Fat	50	**Total Carbohydrate**	21 g
Total Fat	6.0 g	Dietary Fiber	3 g
Saturated Fat	1.3 g	Sugars	16 g
Trans Fat	0.0 g	**Protein**	2 g
Cholesterol	0 mg	**Phosphorus**	55 mg
Sodium	0 mg		

Apricot-Cherry Almond Balls

YIELD: 26 balls

SERVES: 13   SERVING SIZE: 2 balls

PREP TIME: 15 minutes   COOKING TIME: None

Making these treasure troves of sweetness and nutrition is similar to making the Chocolate Walnut Date Balls above, but these treats are for those non-chocolate moments. The dried apricots and cherries provide tons of flavor.

INGREDIENTS ———————————————————————

1 cup raw almonds (5 ounces)

1 cup dried apricots (5 ounces)

1 cup dried tart cherries, sweetened (5 ounces)

1 tablespoon water

INSTRUCTIONS

1   In a food processor, process the almonds on and off for 15–20 seconds or until finely chopped, but not a powder.

2   Add the dried apricots and cherries. Process about 30 seconds at 5- to 10-second intervals or until finely chopped.

3   Add the water and process another 10 seconds to make a sticky mass.

4   Using damp hands, form 26 balls, each weighing about 17 grams.

5   Place the balls in a container with a lid. Separate layers with wax paper. Store at room temperature or the refrigerator.

CHOICES/EXCHANGES
1 Fruit, 1 Fat

BASIC NUTRITIONAL VALUES

Calories	130	**Potassium**	230 mg
Calories from Fat	45	**Total Carbohydrate**	18 g
Total Fat	5.0 g	Dietary Fiber	3 g
Saturated Fat	0.4 g	Sugars	13 g
Trans Fat	0.0 g	**Protein**	3 g
Cholesterol	0 mg	**Phosphorus**	120 mg
Sodium	0 mg		

Menu Ideas

I am no fan of preprinted menu plans because I find that they teach users very little and frustrate them greatly. Why? These preprinted, one-size-fits-all plans contain too much food or too little food, they include disliked or unfamiliar foods, the cooking methods are unfamiliar or too time-consuming, they prevent flexibility or spontaneity, and they include ingredients that are out of season. And there are many more reasons. But I also see the value in sharing ideas. Thus, I'm including a few ideas for each of the three main meals. Let them serve as a guide or inspiration.

Breakfast Ideas

- Greek yogurt with berries and walnuts
- Eggs, mashed avocado, and tomato slices on whole-grain toast; glass of milk
- Peanut butter and banana sandwich on whole-grain bread, glass of milk
- Overnight oats with Greek yogurt, fresh peaches, almonds, and cinnamon
- Low-fat cottage cheese, cinnamon, raisins, muesli

Lunch Ideas

- Nourish Meal Bowl (see pages 156 and 157) with pasta and salmon, strawberries
- Tuna salad with cherry tomatoes, red onion, artichoke hearts, fresh cilantro, and light mayo; whole-grain crackers; apple
- Turkey Taco Soup (see page 144), small tortilla with melted reduced-fat cheese, clementine
- Nourish Meal Bowl (see pages 156 and 157) with quinoa, roasted tofu, and peanuts; fresh berries

- Turkey burger inside a portabello mushroom or on a whole-wheat bun, Chunky Gazpacho (see page 138), pear
- Low-fat cottage cheese mixed with diced tomatoes, fresh basil leaves, and coarse black pepper; whole-grain crackers; orange

Dinner Ideas

- Citrus and Herb Chicken Thighs (see page 142), brown rice, steamed green beans, mixed green salad with Greek Salad Dressing (see page 160)
- Lentil and Sweet Potato Chili (see page 148) topped with strained plain yogurt, mixed vegetable salad with sliced avocado and salsa, glass of milk
- Salmon or favorite fish with Lemon Basil Sauce for Fish (see page 150), roasted potatoes, roasted broccoli (see Roasted Vegetables on page 154), sliced tomato drizzled with extra-virgin olive oil
- Veggie-Heavy Spaghetti Sauce (see page 140), spaghetti, salad with light Italian salad dressing, Apricot-Cherry Almond Balls (see page 166)

Be Empowered

- Select 8–10 random food items in your kitchen. Check the food labels carefully. If they do not contribute to a health-boosting diet, toss them out, give them away, or vow to use them only now and then. Add replacement products to your grocery list.
- Using the shopping guide in this chapter; create a thorough grocery list.
- Think of at least two desserts with benefits that you can enjoy and fit into your balanced diet. Consider something you buy, like chocolate-covered almonds, or something that you make, such as the Mixed Berry Frozen Yogurt in this chapter.
- Add to your healthy recipe library.
- Try out at least one new recipe this week or healthify a favorite recipe.
- Don't forget to share on social media with #LifestyleReset and @NutritionJill.

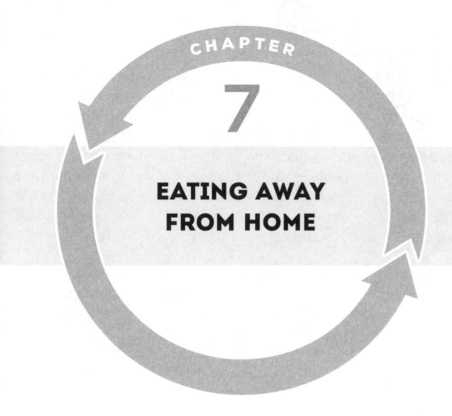

CHAPTER

7

EATING AWAY FROM HOME

*H*ome is where you have the most control over your food choices. With thoughtful planning and consideration, however, you can eat nourishing foods away from home.

Before getting into how to make wise restaurant choices, it's helpful to assess your own eating-out routine or experience. How often do you eat out? Why do you choose to eat out? Would it be helpful to eat out less often, or is making better choices all you really need to do? Think about these questions because they will help you set SMART goals that are pertinent to your lifestyle reset.

13 Restaurant Strategies

The challenges to navigating restaurant meals are many. The portions are often huge. It's hard to know which foods are swimming in sugar and saturated fats. Some foods are sautéed in heart-healthy oils, but others are seared in butter and bacon grease. What sounds like a wholesome wrap or salad may be nothing more than a calorie bomb in disguise. Even if only healthful ingredients come together on your plate, the quantity can eat up your calorie budget in no time. There are a lot of surprises and a lot of unknowns in restaurant meals. The following 13 strategies can help you in any type of restaurant.

1. *Treat it like it's a special occasion only if it's a special occasion.* What was once a treat is now commonplace. Americans eat out much more often than they did a few decades ago. But for many, the idea of splurging when dining out sticks with them even if they visit restaurants a few times each week. Even if they eat out daily! Throwing caution to the wind daily or a few times a week in restaurants is really not moderation and will likely make it hard to meet your health goals. Unless it's truly a special occasion—a wedding anniversary, a birthday, a celebration of a job promotion, or similar event—treat it like any other meal. Try to mimic the portions you eat at home and balance your plate with more nonstarchy vegetables than other types of food.

2. *Make a game plan and stick to it.* Winging it rarely works when it comes to lifestyle changes. So before heading to the restaurant, set your plan. My most successful clients preview menus online and make their choices at home in a leisurely environment. They give themselves time to think through their options instead of being influenced by the orders of dining companions or nudges from the waitstaff. Last-minute choices are frequently less healthful. Check out Healthy Dining Finder (healthydiningfinder.com) to look for restaurants near you that offer healthful fare.

3. *Ask questions.* It's okay to ask questions about how the food is prepared. Ask about the oils or fats used. Stick to heart-healthy liquid oils like canola, olive, and vegetable oils. As much as possible, avoid butter, lard, coconut oil, and bacon grease. Choose leaner cuts of meat such as skinless poultry, baked and broiled fish, and top sirloin steak. Inquire about sauces. Are they rich in fat or added sugars?

4. *Kindly make requests.* A lot of people are too inhibited to make special requests. But my experience is nearly always positive, so I encourage you to make requests too. Consider the following.

   - Can the dish be made with fish instead of beef?
   - Please don't bring bread or chips to the table.
   - Will you ask the chef to use a light hand with the salt?
   - May I have a different vegetable in place of french fries?
   - Will you bring the sauce (or salad dressing) on the side?
   - May I have marinara sauce instead of Alfredo sauce?
   - Please leave the bacon off of my sandwich.

   These questions are not demanding, and your wait staff or the chef should not be offended. The answer might be no, and that means you may need another few minutes to make your selections.

5. *Keep your overall healthy eating plan in mind.* If your plan to go out to dinner includes higher-calorie fare, be mindful earlier in the day to keep calories in check. This doesn't mean that you should starve yourself all day to binge at night. But it is wise to eliminate the extras at other meals. You might eat your lunchtime sandwich without a slice of cheese to save about 100 calories. And you could leave the croutons and ham off your salad. Also think about ways to get in enough fruits and vegetables, two food groups that are frequently lacking from restaurant menus. If you don't think they'll make it to your dinner plate, eat them at earlier meals and snacks.

6. *Manage hunger.* So often I hear advice to eat a snack before heading out to a restaurant or a party. While this is good advice in some situations, it does little more than encourage overeating in other situations. Instead of following blanket advice to eat a snack or not to eat a snack, assess your unique situation. If your meal is likely to be delayed, a small snack is in order. But if you've eaten adequately throughout the day and your meal out is at an appropriate time for you, you likely don't need to pre-eat, and it's probably better not to do so. If you do need a snack, think about what food group is lacking from your diet and go for that. Consider a cup of yogurt, low-fat cheese, a piece of fruit, or any vegetable, including vegetable juice. Once at the restaurant, be sure to order foods that are filling. Start your meal with a low-calorie salad or broth-based soup. Research studies show that this strategy helps to keep calories for the full meal lower.

7. *Be menu savvy.* A few menu descriptors hint that the item isn't prepared in a healthful way. When in doubt, ask your server. Be leery of menu choices with these words: Alfredo, au gratin, batter-dipped, béchamel, breaded, bisque, confit, creamy, crispy, crunchy, crusted, fried, fritters, gooey, golden, rich, roux, scalloped, smothered, sizzling, tempura, or white sauce.

8. *Be aware of health halos of ethnic restaurants.* Many people automatically assume that food in Chinese or Middle Eastern restaurants is light and healthful because these cuisines tend to be rich in vegetables. But often the health halos are undeserved. The food may be prepared in more "American" ways and include much more fat and a larger proportion of meat to vegetables. Even if the food was prepared exactly like it might be in the home country, that doesn't mean that it's light and health boosting. Every type of cuisine has indulgent foods.

9. *Be picky.* Don't eat it just because it's in front of you. If you don't love it, push it aside. Who wants to use up their calorie

budget on food that's mediocre! If you're dining at a buffet, give a good look to everything that's served. The common tendency is to simply start loading up, so the foods at the front of the line tend to fill your plate. Be choosier and more deliberate than that. After scrutinizing the full buffet, select the tastiest and most healthful foods.

10. *Slow down and pay attention.* Focus on every sip and every bite. Taste it. Feel it. Notice the texture, temperature, appearance, flavor, and aroma. It's easy to overeat or eat mindlessly when you're distracted by conversation. Plus, research tells us that our dining companions influence how much and how rapidly we eat. We tend to eat more in large groups. And we tend to eat faster when our companions eat faster. Unfortunately, the faster we eat, the more we tend to eat. Really focus on your speed.

11. *Be portion savvy.* These days, restaurants rarely serve small portions. I typically know that whatever is on my plate is more than I need. Sometimes you can request small portions or order from an appetizer or small plates menu. Ask if you can order a lunch portion at dinner or the appetizer portion instead of the entrée portion. Splitting menu items with a dining companion is commonplace these days, though there is often an additional charge of a few dollars. When your food comes, decide on a proper portion based on the amount you strive to eat at home. Draw an imaginary line through your food, and don't cross that line. Alternatively, you can ask your server to box half your meal before it's brought to the table.

12. *Don't drink your calories.* Sodas, lemonade, sweet teas, and alcoholic beverages can cost you quite a lot of calories—several hundred actually. Be clear on where you want to spend your calorie budget. If it's on food, not drink, order water, unsweetened tea, and the like.

13. *Reconsider the meaning of value.* Once a patient who had made great strides in his lifestyle reset plan—including making

better fast-food choices—told me how he came to order two sandwiches for lunch. He had a coupon for two sandwiches at a reduced price. After weeks of ordering only one sandwich and pairing it with fruit that he brought from home, he ordered two sandwiches simply because of the perceived value. But he actually spent more money than he would have if he had ordered only one sandwich. Plus he got more calories, sodium, saturated fat, and refined grains. It didn't take long for him to realize that he really wasted money and ate up too much of his calorie allowance, all while getting less nutritional value than if he had stuck to the plan of one sandwich and a piece of fruit. Some diners let cost influence their purchases more than any other factor. Other diners feel that they have to get their money's worth by eating everything put in front of them. But there are other, more important, ways to assess value than to consider only the amount of money something costs. Pay attention to health value, nutritional value, and satisfaction value. These things are also important, and they can affect the way you feel immediately after eating and long term. If cost is a major driving factor, choose the least expensive healthful item or share something with a friend. Or take some home to eat again at another meal. Two meals for the price of one is an excellent way to save money and better your health. Instead of cashing in on just any bargain—like two sandwiches for a reduced price—ask yourself if this is truly a good way to spend your money. If you wouldn't buy two sandwiches without the coupon, it's probably not a good idea to buy two sandwiches ever. And finally, instead of feeling wasteful for leaving food, remind yourself that if your body doesn't need the food, you're wasting it whether you eat it or leave it. Overeating is a form of food waste. Ideally, you can freeze leftovers or eat them tomorrow. If not, isn't it better to leave it where it causes no harm—uneaten on your plate?

Better Fare When Eating Out

Use the following guide to make careful choices when eating out. These foods are a recommended sampling of what to order and what to skip. For a very thorough recommendation (more than 500 pages thorough), check out *Eat Out, Eat Well* by Hope Warshaw, published by the American Diabetes Association.

American Fare and Fast Food

Go for It:

- Sandwiches with lean meats such as roast beef, turkey, and chicken (Bulk up your sandwich with extra veggies, not extra meats and cheese. If your bread is very fluffy like a sub roll, you can scoop out and discard some of the doughy part.)
- Salads with lots of colorful veggies, a little dressing, and not much of anything else
- Vegetable soup and other broth-based soups (These soups will fill you up for few calories.)
- Lean meats without creamy or buttery sauces (Try steamed shrimp, grilled tuna, baked salmon, sirloin steak, or baked or rotisserie chicken [without the skin.])
- Steamed vegetables, sliced tomatoes, carrot sticks, fresh fruit, sliced apples
- Fast-food sandwich from the children's menu

Be Careful:

- Croissants and biscuits
- Broccoli-cheese soup, cream of potato soup, and other creamy or cheesy soups
- Deep-fried sides like french fries and onion rings
- Fried chicken or fried fish

- Fatty meats such as prime rib, beef or pork ribs, corned beef, chicken with skin, sausage, bacon, and hot dogs
- Quesadilla
- Large or super-sized sandwiches or burgers (Turkey burgers are frequently made with ground turkey that includes the skin.)
- Fatty sandwich toppings such as bacon, excessive amounts of cheese, fried onions, unknown sauces
- Chicken salad, egg salad, tuna salad (These salads may be very calorie rich because of excessive mayonnaise.)
- Sauces and dressings such as cheese, béarnaise, and hollandaise sauces; gravy; salad dressings (Ask for these items on the side and use the dip-and-stab method. First lightly dip the tines of your fork into the sauce, and then stab your food.)
- Milkshakes

Asian (Specifically Chinese, Japanese, and Thai)

Hint: Use chopsticks to slow you down and to shake off some of the fatty, salty sauces. A good strategy to save calories and money is to order fewer entrees than there are people in your dining party. Three entrees, for example, is usually enough to feed four or five diners.

Go for It:

- Steamed dumplings, steamed spring roll, edamame beans, chicken satay, sushi (government guidelines advise that pregnant women and others with concerns for food safety eat only vegetable sushi or cooked sushi), and seaweed salad
- Miso, wonton, egg drop, hot and sour, and Tom Yum Goong (a Thai spicy, broth-based lemongrass soup with shrimp) soups (But be aware, although these soups are low in calories, most soups are loaded with sodium.)
- Veggie-heavy dishes such as moo goo gai pan, steamed fish with vegetables, and stir-fried meat or tofu and vegetables

- Chicken or salmon teriyaki, Pad Kra Pow (made with a Thai stir-fry basil sauce), and Pad Khing (made with a Thai stir-fry ginger sauce)
- Hot tea
- Fortune cookie (These treats usually provide only about 30 calories.)

Be Careful:

- Fried noodles, egg rolls, chicken wings, spareribs, crab Rangoon, tempura
- Buffets, fast food, and mall fare, where meats are often fried and reheated in extra oil
- Fried dishes like General Tso's chicken and sweet and sour dishes
- Chow mein, fried rice

Breakfast

Hint: American restaurant breakfasts tend to be quite large and rich in highly refined grains. Focus on whole foods and portion control.

Go for It:

- Scooped bagel, which has fewer calories because the doughiest part is scooped and discarded
- Small whole-grain bagel with peanut butter
- Egg sandwich on whole-wheat bread
- Vegetable omelet, scrambled eggs, scrambled egg whites
- Scrambled tofu
- Small side order of pancakes or whole-grain toast
- Yogurt with fruit
- Oatmeal, whole-grain cream of wheat, other whole-grain cereals
- Fresh fruit, 100% fruit juice

Be Careful:

- Croissants, biscuits, coffee cake, cinnamon rolls, pastries, scones, muffins
- Breakfast meats, which tend to be high in saturated fats
- Fried potatoes
- Pancakes, French toast, waffles (These items are usually made with refined flour and are covered with sugary syrups.)
- Ham and cheese omelet, western omelet
- Bagel and cream cheese

Indian

Hint: Ask your server about the types of fats used in various foods. Try to avoid coconut oil and ghee, which is clarified butter. Both are high in saturated fats.

Go for It:

- Papadum, a baked lentil wafer, and chapati, a flatbread
- Lentil soup
- Raita, a combination of yogurt, onions, and cucumbers (Dip your bread in it or enjoy it alone.)
- Dahl (spicy lentils)
- Lean meats, chicken, fish, or shrimp prepared in the following styles: jalpharezi, masala, saag, tandoor, and vindaloo

Be Careful:

- Fried breads such as paratha and poori
- Fried appetizers such as samosa and pakora

- Curries (These dishes are made with coconut milk, which is high in saturated fat.)
- Creamy entrees such as korma and malai

Italian

Hint: Watch out for the portions of pasta in Italian restaurants. A reasonable serving is a single cup or less, but some restaurants load the plate with pasta and add a mere sprinkling of vegetables. If you don't want pasta at all—although there's no reason to avoid a small portion—ask to have your meal served atop a bed of spinach or other vegetable.

Go for It:

- Steamed mussels, clams in tomato sauce, marinated vegetables, prosciutto with melon, caprese salad
- Minestrone and bean soups; stracciatella, which is an egg and vegetable soup
- House salad with dressing on the side
- Tomato-based sauces without cream or fatty meats (Good choices are tomato, pomodoro, marinara, red clam, puttanesca, and cacciatore.)

Be Careful:

- Garlic bread, bread and butter, bread and olive oil
- Fried calamari, fried cheese sticks; antipasti, which is an assortment of meats and cheeses
- Eggplant, veal, and chicken Parmesan, which are floured, fried, and heavy on cheese
- Lasagna, manicotti, and other cheesy, rich casseroles

- Alfredo sauce, which is a mix of butter, cream, and Parmesan cheese, and carbonara sauce, which is rich in fat from eggs, cream, cheese, and Italian bacon

Mexican

Go for It:

- Black bean soup, tortilla soup (hold the bacon and limit the fried tortilla chips); posole, which is a soup or stew made of meat and hominy
- Nopalitos salad, which is made of prickly pear cactus
- Salsa and picante sauce (You don't need to pair salsa with chips. Instead dress your salad with it and spice up tacos, soups, and more.)
- Guacamole (Guacamole contains healthful fats. It's high in calories, so limit the amount you eat.)
- Arroz con pollo, chili, soft tacos
- Fajitas, if you request that the sizzling oil or butter be left off your plate

Be Careful:

- Chips, nachos, chile con queso, quesadilla
- Extra cheese and sour cream
- Deep-fried items like crispy tortillas, salad shells, chili rellenos, chimichangas
- Refried beans, unless they are made without lard

Middle Eastern

Go for It:

- Hummus, baba ghanoush, stuffed grape leaves
- Lentil soup, lemon egg soup, cucumber-yogurt soup

- Tabouli
- Greek salad with dressing on the side
- Shish kebobs
- Kibbeh, which is made with ground meat and wheat; kafta, which is another type of meatball

Be Careful:
- Fried items such as falafel, crispy pita chips, and fried eggplant
- Spanikopita: phyllo dough filled with spinach and feta cheese
- Rich casseroles such as pasticchio and moussaka

Be Empowered

- Determine your eating-out style, and ask yourself what changes will help you reach your eating goals. Set a SMART goal.
- Research your favorite restaurants for healthful menu items. Make a list of good choices, so it will free you of weighing options when you eat out. Keep your list on index cards or in your smartphone.
- Practice eating slowly and with your full attention at home, so it will become second nature even when you eat out.
- Weigh and measure your food now and then at home to help you identify a proper portion when you eat out.

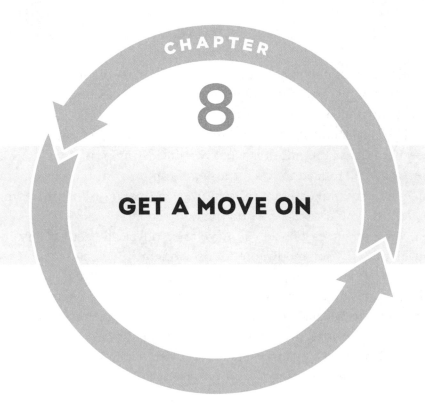

CHAPTER

8

GET A MOVE ON

esearch consistently shows us that physically active people tend to live longer, healthier lives than people who move little throughout the day. Many people think of exercise as the boring or painful drudgery that's required of them to lose weight. And often, when the weight doesn't drop quickly, they quit the exercise. While it's helpful to increase physical activity for weight loss, you will need to exercise *a lot* to see pounds melt off. Even though you may not drop a couple pants sizes by sweating in the gym or walking in your neighborhood after dinner, there are so many reasons to be physically active every day. And it doesn't have to be drudgery!

How Will Exercise Help You?

Exercise is great medicine and great preventive medicine. You already know that regular exercise helps to prevent type 2 diabetes, and that's clearly on your list of reasons to be physically active. Recall that the goal in the Diabetes Prevention Program (DPP) was for participants to exercise at least 150 minutes weekly. Interestingly, regular exercise does not need to lead to weight loss to help prevent type 2 diabetes, since activity makes your cells more responsive to insulin. Every single time you exercise, you do the body good!

What other reasons do you have to be physically active? Just like you identified your motivators to lose weight in Chapter 4, you will benefit from identifying your motivators to exercise. I've created a list below, but it's by no means comprehensive. Again, I've included emotional benefits because these are often just as important as the physical benefits. Go through my list, putting a checkmark next to the benefits that speak to you. Or create a personalized list in your journal or another place where you can refer to it often, especially when your motivation for exercise drops. Add any other motivators you can think of.

- Improve insulin action and blood glucose control
    - Celebrate every exercise session because blood glucose levels improve for 2–72 hours after exercise, depending on the length of time and intensity of your exercise.
- Lower blood pressure
- Raise HDL (good) cholesterol
- Reduce low levels of chronic inflammation
- Lessen risk for type 2 diabetes, prediabetes, metabolic syndrome, heart disease, stroke, diverticulitis, several types of cancer, osteoporosis, overweight, and obesity
- Improve circulation
- Improve sexual function
- Contribute to a healthy brain during aging
- Enhance your immune system

- Contribute to weight management, especially by helping to prevent weight regain
- Boost mood
- Possibly help to prevent or treat depression
- Contribute to a healthy appearance
- Create a sense of accomplishment
- Build self-esteem
- Aid good posture
- Contribute to less pain/more comfort during daily activities
- Help manage stress
- Improve sleep
- Contribute to feelings of energy and vitality
- Strengthen bones, muscles, and joints
- Be a good role model
- Other: _____
- Other: _____
- Other: _____

Exercise Safely

It's common to be very excited and motivated about starting a new exercise plan. But abruptly starting or changing an exercise routine is risky. Slow and steady is the smart way to go to avoid health risks, injuries, and burnout. Before getting started, check in with your health care provider to be certain that you are fit to exercise and to ask for advice about the types of activities that are good choices for you. Both prediabetes and type 2 diabetes are risk factors for heart disease, so this check-in with your health care provider is important. If you take medications for your blood glucose, or should you someday take them, ask about your risk for experiencing hypoglycemia or low blood glucose during physical activity. Fortunately, there are quite a number of medications to lower blood glucose that do not put you at high risk for hypoglycemia.

Exercise Recommendations

You may want to know how much you should exercise and what types of exercise you should do. Before getting into the recommendations, keep a few things in mind.

First, the word *should*, as in how much you should exercise, is anything but empowering. "I should exercise" sounds like it's not a choice and that it's not a desirable thing to do. I prefer more empowering words, so I try to avoid "shoulds" and "shouldn'ts" and reframe my statements when I catch myself saying them. I *choose* to exercise because of the many rewards it brings. It's a subtle difference, but if you practice speaking in positive, empowering language, you'll find you feel more positive and empowered. I promise. Just keep it up. More on that in Chapter 11.

Second, any amount of exercise is better than none! Too many people fail to exercise because they can't find the 30 minutes they think they need. But if they have 15 minutes, they could use it and would surely benefit. If you don't have even 15 minutes, maybe you have 10 or 8 or even 5 minutes. Do you have time to do a few pushups and sit-ups before getting dressed in the morning? If the answer is "yes," do pushups and sit-ups! Sometimes when I have early-morning appointments, I choose to jog around the block instead of jogging my usual 40 minutes. Why? Because every exercise session is good for me and because sticking as closely as possible to my routine makes me feel good and maintain my habit.

Third, you are not like everyone else, so tailor your exercise plan to your likes, needs, and schedule. And as you progress in your exercise plan, you'll find that your needs and likes continue to change, so don't get stuck in an exercise rut or a one-size-fits-all plan.

And finally, you may have specific health concerns, so it's smart to seek the approval of your health care provider before starting a new exercise program.

CDC Exercise Guidelines

To lower the risk of many chronic diseases, the Centers for Disease Control and Prevention (CDC) recommends the following for adults:

- Aim for or build up to at least 150 minutes of moderate-intensity aerobic activity (such as brisk walking) each week *or* at least 75 minutes of vigorous-intensity aerobic activity (such as running) each week.
- Strive to engage in muscle-strengthening activities (such as weight machines and elastic bands) involving all major muscle groups at least twice weekly.
- By doing more, you'll likely experience even greater benefits.

The American Diabetes Association concurs with these general recommendations. The Association adds that for the greatest effects on insulin resistance and for enhanced insulin action, daily exercise is ideal. Aim to have at least no more than two days elapse between exercise sessions.

Components of an Exercise Plan

A complete exercise program includes four types of exercises: aerobic, muscle-strengthening, flexibility, and balance exercises.

Aerobic Exercise

This type of exercise is sometimes called cardiovascular or cardio-respiratory exercise. Aerobic activities use large muscle groups and cause your heart rate to increase and your breath to come faster and more heavily. When you engage in walking, running, biking, swimming, rowing, dancing, jumping rope, cross-country skiing, rollerblading, and many more activities, you are performing aerobic exercise. These activities improve insulin activity, blood vessel function, lung function, and immune function. They help manage weight, lower blood pressure and cholesterol levels, and contribute to feelings of well-being. Now that's a lot to be motivated about!

- Begin at any level you are able. For some people that means a 5-minute walk at a moderate or light intensity, and that's okay. Others are fit to jump into a 60-minute cardio dance class. You should not begin at an intensity more advanced than your abilities. Start slowly and build up.
- Three 10-minutes sessions throughout your day is as adequate as one 30-minute session.
- Work toward engaging in cardiovascular exercise nearly every day with no more than 2 consecutive days without exercise. Gradually increase the length of time of your exercise sessions, the intensity of your exercise, and the frequency of your workouts. But increase just one of these three variables at a time. Aim for at least 150 minutes of moderate-intensity exercise weekly.
- If you are medically able and already fit, you may enjoy high-intensity interval training (HIIT). Please check in with your health care provider before starting this because the intensity of exercise comes with additional risk. HIIT involves short bursts of intense exercise alternated with longer periods of lower-intensity exercise or recovery exercise. An example is alternating 20 seconds of sprinting with 4 minutes of slower recovery jogging.

Muscle-Strengthening Exercise

This type of exercise is also called resistance exercise. Lifting weights, using elastic bands, and lifting your own body weight when performing squats, sit-ups, and pushups are examples of resistance exercises.

These types of exercises increase muscular strength (how much your muscles can lift) and muscular endurance (how long your muscles can exert force). Having both good muscular strength and endurance helps prevent injury. When you build muscle, you boost your metabolic rate. Unfortunately, the effect is small, and many people overestimate the role of weight training on weight loss. Regular strength training increases bone mass and bone strength, helps you maintain independence in activities of daily living as you age, improves insulin sensitivity at least as well as aerobic exercise, lowers blood pressure and cholesterol levels, and improves mental health. A recent study looked at the exercise habits of more than 35,000 healthy women. Compared to women who did no strength training, those who performed strength training exercises were 30% less likely to develop type 2 diabetes and 17% less likely to develop heart disease over an average 10-year follow-up period. The combination of aerobic and muscle-building exercises was associated with an even greater reduction in risk. Again, these are big reasons to be motivated! Unfortunately, a lot of people seem to dismiss the benefits of including strength training and avoid it. Maybe it's not as much fun or perhaps it feels awkward. Try to keep an open mind. Every one of us can benefit.

- Begin at your own pace, but not more than moderate-intensity training. Lift weights or perform an exercise 10–15 times. This is one set of exercises. You are using the right weight if you can perform the exercise properly 10–15 times, but reach the point of failure after that.
- Aim to perform 8–10 exercises targeting different body parts each exercise session.
- Strength train 2 days each week without targeting the same muscle groups two days in a row.
- Progress to heavier weights only when you are consistently able to exceed your target number of repetitions.
- Moderate-intensity training is lifting a particular weight about 15 times and being unable to perform a 16th repetition in good

form. Vigorous intensity is lifting a heavier weight six to eight times before failing.

- When you are ready to progress again, you can increase the number of sets to two or three. Finally, add an additional strength training session for a total of three sessions on non-consecutive days.
- Be certain you are performing the exercise correctly. Lifting a weight that is too heavy will impair your form. It is prudent to work with a skilled certified personal trainer. See Working with a Trainer on page 197.

Flexibility Exercises

Stretching exercises will help you maintain or improve the range of motion of your joints, which can reduce your risk of injury. Joint flexibility tends to decrease with aging, but regular flexibility exercises can improve your range of motion no matter how old you are. Yoga and tai chi include basic stretching movements. Follow these guidelines for safe and effective stretching.

- Stretch warm muscles to reduce the risk of injury. It's smart to warm your muscles by walking around for a few minutes.
- Stretch to the point of tightness or slight discomfort for 10–30 seconds. Increase the length of time as you are able. Repeat for a total of two to four repetitions.
- Perform stretching exercises for all major muscle groups at least twice weekly. Increase the frequency of your stretching sessions as able.

Balance Exercise

Balancing exercises are especially important for older adults because they may help prevent falls. Improving balance can be as simple as practicing standing on one leg, walking backwards, and performing similar exercises several times per week. Yoga and tai chi often combine flexibility, balance, and core-strengthening movements.

- Practice balance exercises at least twice weekly. Progress to more frequent and longer sessions as your skill improves.

Getting Started on an Exercise Plan

As I've already stated, it's a good idea to check in with your health care provider before starting an exercise routine. It's also smart to ease into your program, especially if you've been inactive for some time or if you have a health condition or injury that could get in the way of your progress. Getting into the habit of being active is critical. I feel strongly that developing a solid habit is more important than the immediate physical benefits of exercise. The habit will help you realize those health benefits next month, next year, and all the years after that. To develop the habit, set yourself up to be successful. Create SMART goals (see page 195). I often encourage my clients to build the habit of walking by setting aside at least 5 minutes *every* day rather than longer periods just two or three times weekly. A daily habit is more likely to stick than a sometimes habit. Tiny successes are the building blocks of greater successes, so start small and keep creating slightly more challenging goals.

Determine the Intensity of Aerobic Exercise

Is your exercise moderate or vigorous intensity? For guidance, try one of these measures.

Talk-sing test

If you're engaging in moderate-intensity activity, you can talk easily enough to hold a conversation, but you cannot sing. If you can sing, you are performing light activity. During vigorous-intensity activity, you will not be able to say more than a few words without pausing for a breath.

Heart rate zone

To determine your heart rate zone, you need to know your estimated maximum heart rate, which is your age subtracted from 220. For example, if you are 50 years old, your estimated maximum age-related heart rate is 170 beats per minute (bpm). For example:

220 − age = estimated maximum age-related heart rate

200 − 50 = 170 bpm

You are exercising at a moderate intensity when your heart rate is 50–70% of your maximum heart rate. For example:

50% of maximum heart rate for a 50-year-old person:
$170 \times 0.5 = 85$ bpm

70% of maximum heart rate for a 50-year-old person:
$170 \times 0.7 = 119$ bpm

Thus, a 50-year-old person whose heart rate falls between 85 and 119 beats per minute is exercising at a moderate intensity.

You are exercising at a vigorous intensity when your heart rate is 70–85% of your maximum heart rate. For example:

70% of maximum heart rate for a 50-year-old person:
$170 \times 0.7 = 119$ bpm

85% of maximum heart rate for a 50-year-old person:
$170 \times 0.85 = 144$ bpm

Thus, a 50-year-old person whose heart rate falls between 119 and 144 beats per minutes is exercising at a vigorous intensity.

Calorie burn

According to the CDC, we can also classify exercise as moderate intensity or vigorous intensity based on the amount of calories the body uses per minute of activity.

Moderate Intensity
Walking briskly (3 mph or faster)
Water aerobics
Bicycling slower than
  10 miles per hour
Tennis (doubles)
Ballroom dancing
General gardening

Vigorous Intensity
Race walking
Jogging or running
Bicycling faster than
  10 miles per hour
Tennis (singles)
Swimming laps
Heavy gardening
Jumping rope
Hiking uphill

Measuring Your Heart Rate

To measure your heart rate, stop exercising briefly to take your pulse. Find your pulse on your wrist below your thumb. Place the tips of your index and middle fingers over the artery and press lightly to feel your pulse. Count the beats for 30 seconds and multiply by 2 to determine your heart rate for a full minute. Alternatively, you can count the beats for 60 seconds. Count the first beat as zero and continue counting for the designated time.

Use FITT Principles to Guide Your SMART Goals

The above descriptions of the four components of an exercise plan briefly include guidelines for getting started and progressing.

Use the following FIIT principles to give yourself a more specific plan.

- **F:** Frequency—how often will you do a particular type of exercise
- **I:** Intensity—how vigorously will you exercise
- **T:** Time—how many minutes will you perform the exercise
- **T:** Type—what type of exercise will you do

You can apply the FITT principle to each of the four components of a fitness plan. To build your aerobic fitness, your FITT goal might look like this:

- **F:** at least five times per week
- **I:** at a moderate intensity (At this pace, you can hold a conversation.)
- **T:** for at least 10 minutes
- **T:** dancing (aerobic activity)

Using the above FITT principles, you might create the following SMART goal.

For this week, every weekday (Monday through Friday) after breakfast, I'll dance to lively music in the den for 10 minutes (at a moderate intensity).

This goal is *specific* enough that even a stranger would understand your plan. You know that it's *measurable* because you can identify the number of times you accomplish the goal during the 5-day workweek. Dancing is an *action*. The goal is *realistic* if you are fairly confident that you can achieve it with the resources you have available. Finally, this goal identifies important information about *time*: you will try this goal out for a week and you'll exercise in the time between breakfast and when you get ready to start your day.

As your fitness level improves, you can increase the frequency, intensity, or time. Increase just one of these elements at a time.

Eventually, you can increase all three. Use the FITT principle to plan each component of your fitness program.

Working with a Trainer

There are so many reasons to work with a personal trainer. Many of my patients like the accountability that a trainer provides. If they know that a trainer is expecting them to show up and work out, they're less likely to skip out on a fitness session. A skilled trainer also helps you with motivation and pushes you hard enough without pushing you too hard, which helps prevent exercise burnout and injuries. Everyone can benefit from a personalized fitness program, but anyone with health conditions or a history of injuries is an especially good candidate for working with a trainer.

Choosing a qualified, skilled trainer with whom you can have a good relationship is key.

- Work with a trainer who has been certified by a nationally recognized and accredited certifying organization such as the American College of Sports Medicine (ACSM), the American Council on Exercise (ACE), or the National Academy of Sports Medicine (NASM). Some certifications require very little training and expertise. Be sure to ask enough questions that you are satisfied. Some trainers also have college backgrounds in exercise science, kinesiology, or a related field. Do not take medical advice from a trainer, and do not take nutrition advice unless your trainer is also a registered dietitian nutritionist.
- Hire someone with experience working with people like you—your age, fitness level, health conditions, etc. Ask for references and take the time to check them out.
- Your trainer should ask you about your health history, a previous history of injuries, and your fitness goals. A skilled trainer will customize your program based on a thorough assessment.

- Your trainer should carry professional liability insurance and be trained to perform CPR.
- Ask about the trainer's fees and cancellation policy. Ask if you can share the session and the fee with a friend, if that interests you.
- Chat with a potential trainer to be sure you are a good fit for one another before signing a contract. Even better, find out if you can pay for a single session before agreeing to a long-term program. Do you like this trainer's style? Does the trainer encourage you to work hard or simply tell you what to do and count the reps? Let your trainer know if you like to try new things often or move more slowly. Share all of your concerns.

Make Exercise Fun

Often I hear people say that they hate exercise. To me, this is like saying that they hate food. How could that be? The body is meant to both move and receive nourishment. And just like there are so many types of food, there are so many types of exercise. How could someone hate them all? I suspect that people who say this really dislike the formal exercise programs they have tried in the past. Maybe they find bicep curls and squats difficult and counting reps boring, or they don't like classes in which the instructors sound harsh. Perhaps they don't like the exertion or bouncing that comes with running. When I have conversations with clients about this, it's the rare person who doesn't remember or discover some form of exercise that he or she actually enjoys on some level.

Determine What Specific Part of Exercise You Don't Like

After figuring this out, try to find a solution. Once a client didn't like walking, but it turns out that she didn't have good walking shoes. So what is it exactly that you don't like? Do you feel discomfort or boredom? Do you feel that you look silly? Is your exercise too difficult?

Think Back to Your Childhood

Try an exercise that you enjoyed then. I loved skating, biking with friends, dancing to music, playing tennis, hula hoops, and my pogo stick. Today I mountain bike with my family, play Just Dance on the Wii, and use a weighted hula hoop now and then when I watch TV. Think about what you can bring back into your life.

Start Small

It's better to do less than you are capable of than to do so much that you dislike it and quit. Build your skill at whatever rate is appropriate for you.

Focus on the Habit

That's what really matters. I'd much rather you perform 10 sit-ups a day and build to a long-term habit than start out with bigger goals only to quit next week. Take another look at the section about building habits in Chapter 2. Recall that habits are built more readily when we have some sort of reward. When you finish exercising, reward yourself with some praise. Do that even if it feels a bit silly. Remind yourself that you moved and that it's good for you. Hold on to those thoughts for several seconds or longer.

Match Exercise to Your Personality and to Your Other Goals

If you want more social activity, try a team sport like tennis or bowling or join an exercise class. If you enjoy one-on-one activities, hire a personal trainer, ask a friend to walk or jog with you, or schedule a walk and phone chat with a friend who lives far away. Are you the competitive type? Train for a 5K walk or run. If you like a scavenger hunt or a treasure hunt, try geocaching or use the Pokemon Go app.

Combine Exercise with Other Activities

If you enjoy photography, for example, take photos on scenic walks. If you like TV movies, find an exercise to do in front of the TV. Read while using a treadmill. Listen to an audio book while walking outside, or dance to music in your living room. If you crave new knowledge, listen to Ted Talks or podcasts while working out.

Build Pride

Keep an exercise record to remind yourself of your achievements. One successful client created the type of sticker chart that we often see parents use when their kids are working on new skills. Other clients enjoy sharing their workouts on social media, either by posting directly on social media or sharing with a select group of friends through an app.

Try New Activities

Keep things fresh with new activities. Try out different classes at a gym or yoga studio. Sign up for a self-defense class or ballroom dance lessons. Visit a rock-climbing gym. Join an adventure group that organizes outings. Look for one on meetup.com. If you typically work out inside, take a nature walk or go for a bike ride. Never tried elastic bands or suspension straps like the TRX? Maybe now is a good time. Check out your local library to see the selection of exercise DVDs available to borrow.

Try New Gadgets

No active lifestyle requires gadgets, but let's face it: They're fun. And if a new gadget fits your budget and inspires your lifestyle reset or keeps you on track, then it is money well spent.

- **Pedometer.** A pedometer is perhaps the simplest fitness gadget. Strap it on to your waistband and start walking, and it will keep track of your steps. Be sure to get a reliable one.

Expect to spend $30 or so. A good one will count your steps fairly accurately and will not count every slight move you make. Test it out by taking exactly 100 steps. If your pedometer registers 90–110 steps, it's good enough.

- **Fitness trackers.** These fitness wristbands range substantially in price and function. Expect to pay as little as $50 or as much as a few hundred dollars. I've used the FitBit Flex, which tracks steps, estimates calories burned, sleep, and more. Some fitness bands have a GPS function, track the number of stairs you climb, or measure your heart rate.
- **Heart rate monitor.** Some strap to your chest. Others are worn like a watch on your wrist. The purpose is to help you stay in your targeted heart rate zone during exercise.

Crank Up the Music

The right music can make your workouts more fun and may even make them seem easier. Ideally, the tempo of the music matches the tempo of your activity. Use slower-tempo music for warm-ups and low-impact exercises. Increase the tempo for strength training sessions and even more for faster-paced activities like running and dancing.

Change Your Expectations

Few things make exercise less enjoyable than feeling like a failure. Be realistic. The rewards of exercise are first experienced where we don't see them—inside the body. It takes a long time before we see physical changes.

Picking a Gym

Going to the gym should not feel like drudgery. You should walk into a clean and pleasant place and feel energy. The employees should be friendly and professional, and the gym-goers should look like they're enjoying the experience. Visit the facility during the times you plan to work out. Ask yourself the following questions when looking for a gym.

- Is the location convenient? Using a gym close to work might be good for some, but for many people, a gym close to home is better.
- Are the hours of operation convenient? If you plan to take classes, is the class schedule convenient?
- Do they offer child care? Are the attendants qualified?
- Who is exercising? Does it look like a group with whom you will eventually feel comfortable? If you are a newbie and the gym caters to body builders, it may not be a good fit for you.
- Are the locker rooms, showers, fitness equipment, and exercise rooms clean?
- Are there enough machines available or are people waiting?
- Does it offer the equipment and the exercise experience you want? Is there a four-season pool, racquetball courts, an indoor track, spa facilities, or whatever you want out of your membership?
- Is the staff appropriately trained? Who will teach you how to use the exercise equipment?
- Is there an AED (automated external defibrillator) should someone have a heart attack? Are employees trained to use it? Do they know CPR?
- What do other people say about the facility? Ask a few members what they like or don't like about the facility.
- Can you try out a 1-week membership for free?
- What are the contract terms? Is the cost agreeable to you? Is there an initiation fee? Is there a payment plan? Does the facility have a reciprocal program allowing you to work out in another city for free or a discounted price? Can you put your membership on hold if you're sick, injured, or unavailable?

Be Empowered

- Using the list on pages 186 and 187, identify your motivators to engage in regular physical activity.
- Check in with your health care provider to see if you are free to begin an exercise program or ramp up an existing one.
- Consider the steps necessary to make exercise your habit.
- Using FITT principles, create SMART goals around physical activity. Consider any of the four components of a balanced fitness program.
- Purchase appropriate footwear, clothing, or supplies.

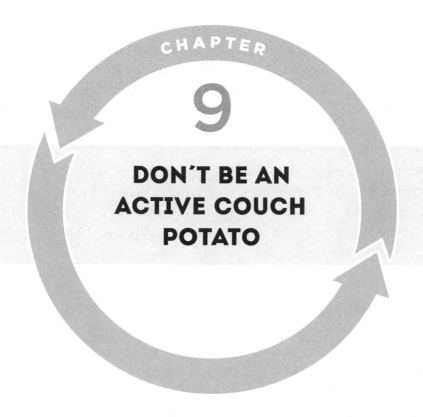

DON'T BE AN ACTIVE COUCH POTATO

*A*lthough it sounds like an oxymoron, it is indeed possible to be an active couch potato. Many people exercise 30 or more minutes daily, but succumb to the comfort of the chair or couch for most of the rest of the day. Although regular exercise is well known to help prevent type 2 diabetes, heart disease, unwanted weight gain, and some cancers, it's rarely enough to overcome an otherwise sedentary lifestyle. The activities of your workday and leisure time matter quite a bit.

Why Are We So Sedentary?

It seems that each decade in recent history brings us more labor-saving devices. We have remote controls to turn on and off the TV and the sprinkler system, adjust the temperature of the house, and light a gas fireplace. We drive to work instead of walking. I find research articles online instead of walking through the library stacks. I load my dishwasher instead of scrubbing my dishes. And I grind coffee in a noisy electric machine instead of using a hand crank. If I'm hungry while driving to work, I don't even have to get out of the car to order, receive, and eat food. Our lives are filled with tools of convenience. But with these conveniences come some disadvantages. While I'm not willing to give up my collection of remote controls, wash dishes by hand, pull the plug on my coffee grinder, or hang up my car keys, I do acknowledge how time-saving and labor-saving devices can potentially harm my health by making me less active, and I look for ways to defeat the draw of inactivity.

How Inactivity Harms

Recall from Chapter 4 that there are three components that combine to make up the total number of calories that you burn each day. Only the physical activity component is greatly within your control. And this portion of the total consists of physical activity for the purposes of getting exercise (like a morning jog or water aerobics class) and activities of daily living as big as walking your dog, tiling your floor, and raking leaves to as little as folding laundry, walking to pick up a ringing phone, and nervously tapping your foot.

Body Weight

It's easy to see that if you spend your days tied to a desk and a computer that you'll burn fewer calories than the worker hauling boxes, trimming trees, or transporting hospital patients by wheelchair. Likewise, if you spend your evenings cleaning house, folding laundry, or playing basketball, you will burn more calories than your friend who is nearly lulled to sleep on the coach by the sound of the TV.

Several years ago, physician and researcher James Levine and his colleagues published research findings suggesting that non-exercise activity plays a large role in body weight regulation. Non-exercise activity thermogenesis (NEAT) refers to the calories burned during movement that is not exercise simply for the purpose of exercise. It's the calories burned when standing, walking to the mailbox, sweeping the floor, letting the dogs in and out, repairing a backyard deck, planting a garden, and so on. Some people burn a lot of calories through non-exercise activity. Others, not so much. Week after week and year after year, these calories that are either being burned or not can make a significant difference to your weight and your health.

For 10 days, Levine and colleagues measured the movements of 20 volunteers who described themselves as couch potatoes. None were gym-goers or participated in exercise for the purpose of being physically active. The researchers fitted 10 lean participants and 10 participants with mild obesity with devices that measured their posture and movements twice every second. On average, the participants with obesity sat for an additional 2 hours per day compared to the lean participants. According to the researchers, if the individuals with obesity had copied the non-exercise activities of the lean subjects, they would have burned an extra 350 calories daily, enough to make significant differences in their weights over time. So even without purposeful exercise, the leaner subjects burned more calories because of their NEAT-enhanced behaviors like standing, fidgeting, and moving during daily activities.

Beyond Body Weight

Sedentary behavior is any activity other than sleeping that occurs in a sitting or reclining posture and burns little calories. High amounts of sitting and other sedentary behaviors are associated with poorer health outcomes, even among regular exercisers. In one study, healthy, physically active adults who watched the most TV had larger waist sizes, higher blood pressure levels, and worse blood glucose levels. Researchers find links between the amount of sitting and the risks of developing type 2 diabetes, heart disease, and some types of cancer. In general, as sitting increases, so do the risks of disease and death.

The reasons may be related to weight as described above, but also to other metabolic problems. For example, even among healthy volunteers with normal blood glucose levels, cutting daily steps from more than 10,000 to less than 5,000 for a mere 3 days led to greater blood glucose spikes after eating. Some scientists speculate that prolonged inactivity leads to the suppression of some muscle enzymes, which may result in worsening cholesterol and triglyceride levels. Additionally, when we fail to contract our muscles, less glucose exits the blood to enter the muscle cells.

Take Movement Breaks

Interestingly, taking small breaks from sitting or other sedentary behavior is beneficial. The American Diabetes Association recommends avoiding long periods of sedentary behavior. The Association advises us to break up long periods of sitting with 3-minute breaks every half hour to improve blood glucose control. If you have a sitting job, it may take some creativity to find ways to be less sedentary. In those 3 minutes, you could walk to the bathroom and back, walk in place, do pushups against the wall, do lunges and squats, or any activity that suits you.

Identify Your Patterns of Activity and Sedentary Behavior

Adults under age 60 years of age spend about 6–8 hours daily in sedentary behavior. Older adults are sedentary 8.5–9.6 hours each day. There are many cues to sitting—chairs in a waiting room, desk chairs, or comfy TV chairs. Certainly, we are influenced by the company we keep. If we spend time with sitters, we too are likely to be sitters. But if our friends and family take walks, shoot hoops, dance, and participate in other active leisure-time activities, we are more inclined to do the same.

People often tell me that they are so busy during the day—even if their busyness is a type of sedentary busyness—that they don't have energy left at the end of the day to do anything active. They are drawn to the chair immediately after finishing their daytime chores and stay there until bedtime. Isn't it odd that sitting all day is tiring? I find this when I travel by car or plane and when I'm stuck in a doctor's waiting room for a couple of hours. I've also seen, fortunately, that just a little bit of activity spurs on interest in more activity. When my clients fight the lure of the chair to take a walk or do something active, it nearly always results in so many positive effects that some form of activity eventually becomes the preferred behavior. Isn't it interesting that we can fight fatigue by being active?

Spend some time thinking about why and how you engage in sedentary activities. If you have a pedometer or an accelerometer-type fitness tracker, you can learn your baseline activity levels fairly simply. Strap on your device and let it measure your movement. Keep a record for a few days to a week. If you find that you're not active enough, set a SMART goal to increase your daily steps by 500 or 1,000. Once that pace is comfortable, add another 500–1,000 steps to your daily goal. Aim to eventually accumulate at least 10,000 steps daily. Many devices don't identify periods of activity and inactivity, so looking at the total steps per day may not help you break up periods of sedentary behavior. A tracking sheet like the one on the next page can help you. You can use the blank Activity/Inactivity Record in Appendix B on page 281.

In the example, a woman tracked her activities for a full day and made a note of the amount of active or standing time. Each activity block in which she was active for less than 3 minutes in a 30-minute period is circled. While it isn't feasible or even smart to be

Activity/Inactivity Record

Record your activities throughout the day. Make note of when you stand, walk, or otherwise engage in activity. Keep records for a few days, including both weekdays and weekends. Identify each block of time in which you are inactive, defined as less than 3 minutes of activity in a 30-minute period.

Day: _Monday_   **Date:** _February 20_

Time	Activity	Minutes Active or Standing/Total Minutes
6:00–6:20 A.M.	Wake up, drink coffee, read email	3/20
6:20–6:45 A.M.	Prepare and eat breakfast, pack lunch	4/25
6:45–7:45 A.M.	Jogging and strength training	60/60
7:45–8:20 A.M.	Shower and dress for work	25/35
8:20–9:00 A.M.	Drive to work, arrive to desk	(2/40)
9:00 A.M. to 12:00 P.M.	Work at desk, bathroom break	(3/180)
12:00–12:30 P.M.	Lunch break	6/30
12:30–3:00 P.M.	Work at desk, bathroom break	(3/150)
3:00–3:10 P.M.	Walking break	10/10
3:10–5:30 P.M.	Work at desk, bathroom break	(3/140)
5:30–6:15 P.M.	Walk to the car, drive home, arrive home	(3/45)
6:15–7:15 P.M.	Greet family, change clothes, prepare dinner	60/60
7:15–7:45 P.M.	Eat dinner	(0/30)
7:45–8:30 P.M.	Household and family chores	35/45
8:30–10:30 P.M.	Watch TV and read	(0/120)
10:30–10:45 P.M.	Get ready for bed	15/15
10:45 P.M.	Go to bed	–

active while driving to and from work or while eating dinner, there are four activity blocks that are ideal for her to take active breaks. She is inactive during three long blocks of time while working at her desk and again for 2 hours while relaxing with the TV or a book before bed. With this awareness, she can make goals for active breaks both during the workday and at home. After brainstorming solutions, she might choose several of the following ideas. More ideas are in the next section.

At work:

- Stand up each time she sips water, coffee, or tea
- Stand up each time the phone rings
- Walk to coworkers' desks instead of calling or emailing
- Set a timer to remind her at regular intervals to do toe raises, squats, and pushups against the wall

At home:

- Relax with active activities instead of sedentary activities
    - Walk, play active videogames, play catch with the kids
- Walk, stretch, squat, or lunge during TV commercials
- Stand during TV credits
- Walk for 3 minutes after reading one chapter

Boosting NEAT

Depending on what you find from your activity assessment, you may want to engage in more active leisure-time activities like taking a ballroom dance class, gardening, or leisurely riding your bike after work. Or you may want to focus on breaking up sedentary behavior with short bouts of movement. Or perhaps you'll do both. If you are very inactive, it's probably wise to start with breaking up excessive sitting. Then move on to active leisure activities, and finally, move on to planned exercise.

Try some of these ways to be less sedentary.

- Use a treadmill desk. This is my favorite strategy. In fact, I'm writing the majority of this book while walking 1.5 miles per hour. Fortunately, I have ample space in my home office. I completely get that most people don't have this option.
- Greet visitors to your office. I do this in my patient office. I bring each patient from the waiting room to my office at the start of our appointment time and walk each person out at the end. This ensures that I get up from my desk regularly.
- Use the stairs instead of the elevator.
- Walk to the bathroom farthest from you.
- Ask coworkers to join you for a walk-and-talk meeting.
- Walk the long way to a coworker's desk or to the office kitchen.
- Talk to coworkers in person instead of using the phone and emails.
- As you move from one type of task to another, take a 3-minute activity break.
- Do squats, toe raises, or wall pushups while reheating your coffee.
- Let your dog in and out instead of asking a family member to do it.
- Walk in place or do sit-ups during TV commercials.
- Take 3-minute walk or dance breaks after 30 minutes of reading, studying, paying bills, and other sitting activities.
- Watch TV while using a hula hoop, treadmill, or stationary bicycle.
- Take the dog for a walk.
- Play with your kids or grandkids or even with your neighbor's kids.
- Carry items upstairs or from the car one at a time.
- Walk while talking on the phone.
- Park far from the entrance of a store, office, or friend's home.
- Walk the golf course instead of riding.
- Walk on the beach or toss a Frisbee instead of sitting.

- Choose a different family outdoor activity every weekend. Try hiking, biking, visiting a farmer's market, walking on the beach, playing croquet, swimming, roller skating, visiting a petting zoo, etc.
- Take a 15-minute walk after eating.

Makes Cues to Be Active

Just like we have cues to sit, you can use cues to get yourself more active. If you want to use your stationary bike or treadmill at home, get it in working condition and move it to a room where you'll both see it and use it. If you spend your days at home, lace up athletic shoes to make movement more comfortable and more likely. If you want to be active after work, dress in athletic clothes once you get home. Schedule a dance class or a walk with a friend, so you know that someone is expecting you. If you want to add a few minutes of exercise into your day, simply spreading out a yoga mat or moving hand weights onto the floor earlier in the day might do the trick.

Be Empowered

- Commit to limiting sedentary activities.
- Assess your leisure-time and work-time sedentary behavior by using a step counter or the Activity/Inactivity Record in Appendix B (on page 281), or both.
- Select five ways to break up sedentary behavior at home and work.
- Select at least one active leisure activity to replace an inactive leisure activity.

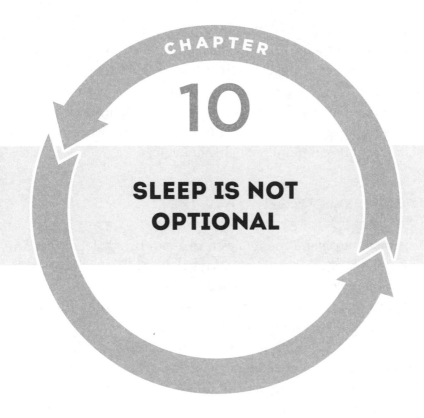

CHAPTER

10

SLEEP IS NOT OPTIONAL

S leep is not a luxury; it is a necessity. And "getting by" on
6 hours of sleep nightly is not getting by unscathed. Sleep loss
causes harm, including possibly bumping up the risk of developing type 2 diabetes. For many of us, when we're extra busy, sleep
is the first thing we cut.

For lots of people, getting adequate sleep is the hardest part
of their lifestyle reset, and that's because of their long-held belief
that sleeping takes time away from things that are more important
or more fun. I felt that way for many years when my children were
little. I started my workday much too early, so I could be available when
they returned home from school. Even though I frequently wished that
it were possible to inject caffeine directly into my tired, foggy brain,
I naively believed that being sleep-deprived was about nothing more
than discomfort. I had no idea the harm I was causing myself.

Oddly, some people even wear lack of sleep, especially losing sleep from being busy, as a badge of honor. Getting adequate Zs, however, is no less important than eating wholesome foods, being physically active, and maintaining a healthful weight. In fact, regular shut-eye may have a direct impact on our weight, and it certainly affects our energy, motivation, and focus for the work involved in developing and maintaining healthful habits.

What Happens During Sleep

We are meant to spend about one-third of our lives asleep! The American Academy of Sleep Medicine says that adults should get at least 7 hours of sleep nightly. Sleeping is a very productive time that greatly affects the other two-thirds of our lives. Yet, according to the CDC, 23% of adults report sleeping only 6 hours per day, and 12% report getting a mere 5 hours or less. In recent decades, the percentage of adults suffering from inadequate sleep has grown considerably.

Some aspects of sleep are still a mystery, although clearly sleep affects how we feel, look, and perform. It appears that sleep is critical for many normal functions including optimal learning, holding on to memories, rest and recovery of muscles, optimal release and balance of hormones, repair of organs, and adequate immune function. All of these things require actual sleep, not just rest.

It's not only the *quantity* of slumber that affects our well-being. Sleep *quality* is also critically important. In a recent report, the National Sleep Foundation recommends that good sleep quality involves being asleep at least 85% of the time that you're in bed, falling asleep within 30 minutes of going to bed, awakening for more than 5 minutes only one time nightly or not at all (twice nightly for older adults), and being awake for a total of no more than 20 minutes after initially falling asleep.

There are two basic categories of sleep: rapid eye movement (REM) sleep and non-REM sleep. Non-REM sleep, which accounts for about 75% of your total sleep, includes the deep sleep in which your body rests and recovers. The other 25% of sleep is REM sleep, in which the brain is active in the work of learning and memory. During REM sleep is typically when you dream as well. During a night of good slumber, you will likely go through the stages of sleep about five times—non-REM sleep, then REM sleep, and repeat four times.

Take a Nap

The National Sleep Foundation recommends that sleepy individuals nap for 20–30 minutes to increase alertness and to reduce mistakes and accidents. They recommend avoiding naps close to bedtime when possible, to reduce the likelihood that a nap will disrupt longer periods of sleep.

Effects of Poor Sleep

With this knowledge, it's not hard to understand that inadequate sleep causes many problems. Among other things, not sleeping enough can lead to daytime sleepiness, mood disturbances, inability to pay attention, cognitive impairment, driving accidents, inadequate growth in children and teens, and a greater risk of chronic health problems.

Obesity

Typically, sleeping too little is associated with gaining more weight. In one study, women who slept only 5 hours per night gained more weight over 16 years than women who slept 6 hours nightly, and those women gained more weight than women who slept 7–8 hours nightly. Adequate sleep helps to maintain a normal balance of appetite hormones.

When sleep is poor or short, the levels of ghrelin, a hunger hormone, go up. And the levels of leptin, a hormone that makes us feel full, go down. Not surprisingly, those changes in appetite hormones can lead to poor eating habits. Researchers noted that when men and women of a healthy weight were sleep-deprived, they ate several hundred calories more than when they were allowed to sleep normally. Short sleeping especially leads to more high-fat foods and snacks.

Diabetes

As weight goes up, so does the risk of developing prediabetes and type 2 diabetes. But inadequate sleep may affect diabetes risk beyond its role in weight gain. The balance of growth hormone and cortisol may also be important. Too little sleep and poor-quality sleep affect glucose metabolism. Researchers in the Netherlands found that restricting sleep to 4 hours a night decreased insulin sensitivity by 20–25% compared to sleeping 8.5 hours a night. When scientists reviewed several studies, they found that people who slept 7–8 hours per day had the lowest risk of type 2 diabetes.

Heart Disease

Both weight gain and disturbances in glucose metabolism affect the risk of developing heart disease. Too little or poor sleep likely affects the chances of developing heart disease in additional ways such as causing problems with blood pressure and increasing low levels of inflammation.

Get a Better Night's Sleep

Sound slumber is such a challenge for so many people. Like any other part of your lifestyle reset, examine what you're doing well (don't neglect this important part), what you could do better, and set some goals. Here are 13 tips for a better night's sleep.

Obstructive Sleep Apnea: A Special Concern

Obstructive sleep apnea is a disorder in which an individual stops breathing momentarily during sleep because the upper airway collapses. These pauses in sleep may occur as many as 100 times per hour. Sleep apnea may result in periods of too little oxygen in the blood, non-restful sleep, inflammation, insulin resistance, an increase in the risk of type 2 diabetes and heart disease, as well as other problems. Not only does obstructive sleep apnea boost the risk of developing type 2 diabetes, but research also suggests that having type 2 diabetes increases the risk of developing sleep apnea. The good news is that treatment for obstructive sleep apnea can improve insulin sensitivity and glucose metabolism in many patients.

Symptoms of obstructive sleep apnea include loud snoring, episodes of not breathing during sleep (observed by another person), excessive daytime sleepiness, morning headaches, and awakening with a dry mouth or sore throat. Obstructive sleep apnea is more likely to affect you if you are male, have a thick neck, smoke, have obesity, use alcohol or sedatives, or have a family history of the sleep disorder. Treatments include weight loss, avoiding alcohol and tobacco, changes in sleeping positions, surgery, and a nighttime breathing device called continuous positive airway pressure (CPAP). In a study of people with prediabetes, using CPAP improved measures of insulin sensitivity.

1. *Help your circadian rhythms.* Circadian rhythms are the physical and mental changes that follow a near 24-hour cycle and respond primarily to light and darkness. Among other things, circadian rhythms affect sleep-wake cycles. Light stimulates a part of the brain that affects our feelings of wakefulness and drowsiness. Thus, exposing yourself to light during the day and decreasing light exposure at night helps to maintain your body's natural rhythms. When you

get up in the morning, open the blinds to allow the light to get you started on your day. First light stimulates the release of the hormone cortisol, raises your body temperature, and inhibits the release of melatonin, the hormone that invites sleep. Shift workers often have trouble because their schedules oppose their circadian rhythms. Visit the National Sleep Foundation website (nationalsleepfoundation.org) for tips, and talk to your health care provider for specific advice. When possible, scheduled naps during shift work are beneficial.

2. *Mind the light at night.* Avoid light from TV, tablets, and computers shortly before bed because these lights are enough to stimulate you and thwart an easy slumber. Keep your room dark for sleeping too. Use blackout blinds to block light from outside. If you need a light in the middle of the night, shine a low illumination nightlight in your hallway or bathroom. Turn your clock away or dim its light. If someone else must leave a light on, go to bed with an eye mask.

3. *Create a routine.* The National Sleep Foundation recommends getting to bed and waking up approximately the same time each day, even on weekends. To ease yourself into bed and into sleep, establish a soothing nighttime ritual such as reading (not on a tablet, computer, or phone), meditating, practicing yoga, sipping on hot decaffeinated tea, or listening to relaxing music.

4. *Cool off.* A cool room can help you get a more sound sleep. Experts recommend dialing down the temperature to a cool 60–67°F. A warm bath or shower before bed may help too because it will first raise your body temperature and allow you to feel sleepier when your body temperature drops in your cooler bedroom.

5. *Silence the noise.* If noises disturb you, block them with earplugs, a fan, or a white noise machine.

6. *Get comfy.* Maybe it's time for a new mattress, sheets, or pillow. Or maybe it's time to send your pets or children to their own beds. A cluttered bedroom may also make you uneasy at night.
7. *Don't fret.* Instead of lying in bed watching the clock and worrying about losing Zs, relax with deep breathing exercises or meditation. If that doesn't send you to sleep, get out of bed for a short time to read or listen to soothing music.
8. *Be active every day.* Regular exercise means more sleep and a sounder slumber.
9. *Avoid caffeine.* This stimulant increases alertness and can cause insomnia. Although it combats daytime sleepiness, it might be the cause of nighttime wakefulness. One study found that consuming caffeine as early as 6 hours before bed hindered good sleep. However, people vary in the length of time it takes to metabolize caffeine, so some people will need to avoid it for much longer than 6 hours before heading to bed.
10. *Eat wisely.* Avoid large meals for 3 or so hours before bed. If you're hungry before bed, eat a very small snack.
11. *Drink wisely.* Alcoholic beverages may push you into sleep faster, but they will also wake you up sooner and more often. Alcohol might interfere with circadian rhythms, block REM sleep, increase snoring, and send you to the bathroom frequently.
12. *Avoid nicotine.* It's a stimulant.
13. *Talk with your health care provider.* If you lose sleep more than just occasionally, seek help from your health care provider. You may have a sleep disorder or an underlying medical condition that affects your sleep. Treatments are available. If you are waking up frequently to urinate, you may have diabetes. High blood glucose may be the reason you need to visit the bathroom often.

Be Empowered

- Identify your motivators to get enough sleep and to sleep soundly. Think of both short- and long-term benefits of good sleep. Jot them down in your journal.
- Ask yourself, are you are pleased with the quantity of your sleep? The quality of your sleep? If not, commit to getting adequate sleep. Review the 13 tips to getting a better night's sleep, and implement one or more strategies.
- If you wonder if you have sleep apnea, another sleep disorder, or a medical condition that affects your sleep, make an appointment with your health care provider.
- If after implementing strategies for better sleep, you are still not sleeping soundly or long enough, discuss your sleep habits with your health care provider.

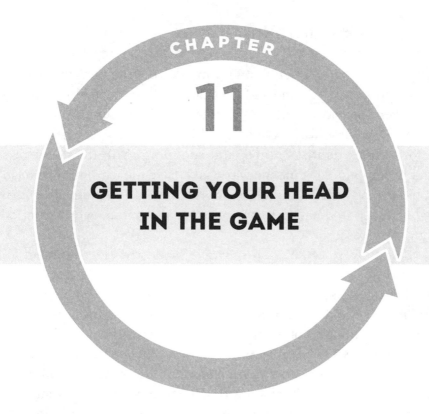

CHAPTER

11

GETTING YOUR HEAD IN THE GAME

*M*any of us reach for salty, rich, gooey, or sugary foods when we feel hurt, sad, mad, lonely, or aggravated. Eating in times of stress may numb you, soothe you, calm you down, or help you avoid your feelings—at least temporarily. An unwelcomed side effect is that emotional eating usually delays or prevents us from reaching our health goals. And it does next to nothing to help us effectively deal with whatever is bugging us. Other head traps, like perfectionism and "catastrophyzing," similarly stall progress. If you're frequently frustrated with yourself for overeating, eating poorly, or not exercising, the solution may lie in your thought processes and the words you say to yourself. There are many obstacles to healthful eating and living. Fortunately, we can actually do something about the obstacles that are our thoughts.

Meet Your Autopilot

Recently, I meant to take a 20-minute drive straight down a single street to meet my husband and dogs for a walk on a beautiful trail one town over. Instead, I turned right after several minutes and kept on driving—the same way I go to my office, grocery store, hairdresser, doctor's office, dentist's office, and shopping mall. It's no surprise that my autopilot took me the way that I drive most often. Who hasn't done this many times! Our autopilots do much more than direct driving behaviors and eating behaviors. Our autopilots even direct our thought processes.

Being aware of habitual negative or destructive thoughts and purposefully working to halt them can be a game-changer during your lifestyle reset. Over the years, hundreds, if not thousands, of patients have told me stories about spiraling downward because of exaggerated thoughts of doom, desperation, or self-loathing.

The following example, unrelated to a lifestyle reset, may help to make this concept clearer. Imagine that you sent a friend a very thoughtful birthday gift, but you didn't get an acknowledgment. You might think that your friend is mad at you or didn't find your gift thoughtful at all. These thoughts can lead to more negative thoughts and still more negative thoughts and, in extreme cases, even affect your feelings of self-worth. In reality, maybe your friend is out of town or your thank you is lost in cyberspace or a thoughtful acknowledgment is on the way. Your friend might even be dealing with a grave crisis or a great celebration that has taken attention away from your kind gesture. The truth is, you just don't know. But allowing the negative response to take hold can push you on a downward spiral. The same is true with your automatic thoughts about your efforts with diet, exercise, sleep, and any other part of your reset. Tanya felt guilty about eating a cookie, so she ate five more since "she's never able to stick to any plan anyway and is doomed to be fat." Automatic negative self-talk has a terrible way of making us feel worse about ourselves and holding us back. Negative self-talk does not push us forward.

Thoughts are not facts. Thinking that your friend is mad at you is not proof that your friend is mad at you. Eating a cookie is not evidence that you are doomed to being overweight. Yet so often, we internalize our thoughts as facts, and we act on them as if they are facts. But *thoughts are not facts.* If you've struggled with your weight or with healthful lifestyle behaviors, chances are quite good that you've beaten yourself up over less-than-stellar choices or negative outcomes. It's likely that you've allowed your autopilot to repeat hurtful words inside your head. Take a few moments to play back some of your thoughts when you didn't live up to your own diet and health expectations. Were you kind to yourself or hard on yourself? Did you truly assess your situation or allow your autopilot to take over? Here is a very common example of stories I hear in my office.

Mary is a busy mom trying to eat better and manage her weight as part of her strategy to prevent type 2 diabetes.

Scenario: I came home from taxiing the kids all over the place and dealing with a mess of traffic only to find that my dog chewed up one of my new throw pillows. I was exhausted, irritated, and angry.

Behavior: I headed straight to the Halloween candy that I bought to give out next week and ate at least four pieces of candy, maybe more. Since I ate so fast, I don't really know.

Negative Self-Talk: Well I blew it again. I'm such a pig! And I'm so weak! I'll never lose weight because I have no self-control, and I'm doomed to get diabetes.

Reaction: I screwed up my diet, so I really went for it! Instead of preparing the healthy meal I planned, I had my husband pick up greasy fried chicken and tater tots. Then I didn't even take my after-dinner walk.

In this story, the automatic feelings of disgust and self-doubt took Mary into a deep downward spiral. She automatically thought that she is weak, has no self-control, and is doomed to develop type 2 diabetes. These thoughts are not facts, even though she has likely said them to herself many times before. While it is true that in this story Mary did not exercise great self-control, it is not a fact that she has no self-control. There are, in fact, many examples in her life—even recent life—where she exercised extreme self-control. And it is certainly not a fact that she will never lose weight and is doomed to get diabetes.

In his excellent book, *The Now Effect*, mindfulness expert Elisha Goldstein, PhD, describes the space between a stimulus and response as a choice point. Mary's autopilot can tell her that she is weak and that she will never lose weight and is doomed to get diabetes. Or Mary can learn to become aware of her automatic thoughts and behaviors and make a choice about them. She can choose to let herself believe that thoughts are facts. She can choose to allow herself to believe that she is a weak person and that she has no self-control. She can give in to the belief that she'll surely develop diabetes. Or she can take notice of these harmful, automatic thoughts and recognize that they are not facts. Take a look at how the same scenario might have played out differently if Mary had recognized one or more of her choice points, the space between the stimulus and her reaction.

Scenario: I came home from taxiing the kids all over the place and dealing with a mess of traffic only to find that my dog chewed up one of my new throw pillows. I was exhausted, irritated, and angry.

Behavior: I headed straight to the Halloween candy that I bought to give out next week and ate at least four pieces of candy, maybe more. Since I ate so fast, I don't really know. (Mary's behavior is still on autopilot, and so are her thoughts, as you see next.)

Negative Self-Talk: Well I blew it again. I'm such a pig! And I'm so weak! I'll never lose weight because I have no self-control, and I'm doomed to get diabetes.

At this point, she works with her choice point and prevents her autopilot from dictating her thoughts.

> *Reaction:* Actually . . . there are a gazillion times I've shown self-control—even yesterday when I ate only one bite of birthday cake at Lauren's party. Tearing into the bag of Halloween candy isn't getting me closer to my goals. I'll stick to my plan for dinner, really watch my portions, focus on enjoying my after-dinner walk, and tomorrow I'll bring out my food record again to help me stay accountable to myself.

Stopping her autopilot and working with her choice point allowed her to avoid the downward spiral of self-loathing and continued poor eating behaviors. She was able to recognize that her thoughts of never being able to lose weight and being doomed to a diagnosis of diabetes were not facts. Our days are filled with choice points. And we can learn to recognize them and respond in more helpful ways. I use the three-step process below to work with automatic negative thoughts. But if you really struggle with them, working with a psychotherapist is a smart strategy, as is practicing mindfulness. *The Now Effect* is a very good guide to make mindfulness practical.

Three-Step HOP to Stopping Negative Self-Talk

1. **H:** Hear your words in your head. Taking this step might be the hardest part because we are habitual in our thoughts and reactions. You may already be on a downward spiral once you hear your negative self-talk. Start from whatever point that you hear yourself. As you work on this, you will be able to catch yourself earlier in the process.
2. **O:** Observe the situation objectively, as if you were observing a friend. Most likely, you'll see that the words are too harsh for

the situation. Draw on your compassion and think about what you would say to your friend.

3. **P:** Plan how to proceed. This plan might include ways to direct your attention to different things, ways you can navigate a similar situation in a better way next time, or ways to reaffirm your commitment to your lifestyle reset.

Kindness First

Once a client told me that she uses a cardio machine at the gym for exactly 47 minutes because that's how long it takes to burn a certain number of calories, and she "has to do that" since she had gained weight recently. I think it's great that she developed a regular workout schedule. What bothered me was the way she came to this routine. And never mind that cardio machines are notoriously wrong at determining a user's calorie burn. In conversation, I learned that she felt desperate about her weight. She was mad at herself and mad at her body—all common emotions I've heard many times. She forced this exercise routine on herself because she believed she deserved this form of punishment. She was acting with a punitive mindset instead of a kindness mindset. There are lots of good reasons to exercise, just as there are lots of good reasons to eat healthfully. But punishing yourself isn't one of them.

I ask my clients to make their food, exercise, and other lifestyle decisions from a place of kindness. Instead of thinking, "I'm fat. I have to exercise," practice saying to yourself, "I *choose* to exercise because I feel great afterward and it's good for my body." Or perhaps you'll say, "I *choose* not to go to the gym today because it's good to take a day off now and then," instead of saying, "I'm not going to the gym today because I'm lazy and I'll always be fat." If you practice this kindness mentality, it too will become habit. It will become your autopilot. It may take a while, but I'm certain that you'll be much happier for it. You'll feel less desperate and have less guilt and anger at yourself. You'll feel more in control. Plus, those healthy habits you're working on are much more likely to sink in when you nudge yourself with a carrot instead of whack yourself with a stick.

10 Common Mind Traps That Stall Progress

Here are an additional 10 mind traps that might hold you back. Some are likely a result of your autopilot, so push that autopilot aside and work to respond in more helpful ways. Others are simply irrational ways of thinking.

1. *Justification*. "I deserve this junk food or I deserve several cocktails because I've been working so hard."

   In reality, how much effort you put into your work and what you eat and drink are unrelated.
2. *All-or-nothing thinking*. "Since I didn't stick to my plan at lunch, I might as well pick up a couple of candy bars. I can start fresh tomorrow."

   This is as logical as choosing to buy furniture you can't afford because you overspent on clothing. After all, you can start fresh with your finances another time. It's much smarter to forgive your indiscretion and move on.
3. *Perfectionism*. "I won't let chocolate pass my lips until I lose 35 pounds."

   Unrealistic rules often lead to diet failure by way of self-loathing or all-or-nothing thinking. Because it's impossible to keep a perfect diet, it's more reasonable to aim for a very good diet. Some of my clients find it helpful to aim for a diet that's at least 80% perfect, but to do that 100% of the time. This puts the focus on a diet that's good enough but reminds them of the importance of being consistent. After all, what we do most of the time is more important than what we do every once in a while.

4. *Ignoring the positive and exaggerating the negative.* "I can't believe that I ate three fried appetizers at the party."

This is similar to seeing the glass half empty. Many of my clients come in to my office feeling like they need to confess their diet and exorcise sins. So while they're telling me of the "bad" things they did, I'm hearing the positive things they also did. For example, the person who ate fried appetizers passed up cocktails and dessert. I'd much rather hear her start the story with these fantastic things, so she feels empowered by the new skills she's developing.

5. *"Catastrophyzing."* "I ate cake at the office party. I'll never be good at my diet."

Don't allow your mind to interpret negative things as disasters. Slipping up on your diet plan doesn't make you a failure at healthful eating any more than knocking into your neighbor's garbage can on collection day means that you're a menace on the road. To put your situation into perspective, ask yourself if this diet or exercise slipup will really matter in the long run. Will it matter in 3 months? In 3 weeks? In 3 days? Chances are pretty good that nothing you ate, any exercise session you missed, or any bedtime goal you failed to meet will matter if you allow yourself to get back on track and move on. These things typically matter only when we allow them to become bigger than they truly are, which is demoralizing and holds us back.

6. *Focus on unfairness.* "It's so unfair that my workout partner does the same workouts I do, but looks so much fitter."

It might seem unfair that some people respond more readily to exercise or seem not to struggle with their weight. In reality, fairness has nothing to do with it.

7. *Different rules apply to thin people.* "Since my husband is thin, I asked him to keep the leftover birthday cake away from me by eating all of it."

The truth is that a lot of birthday cake (pizza, chips, cookies, fill in your favorite "taboo" food) is good for no one—overweight or not—and a small piece rarely hurts anyone—overweight or not. I'd rather see the cake in the freezer or even the trash than have it pushed onto a thin person. Thin people need a balanced diet rich in fruits, vegetables, and other wholesome foods just like people who aren't thin. And thin people with poor diets are also at risk for many chronic diseases.

8. *Social comparisons.* "I should be able to cook dinner every night because my coworkers all do."

    Whether it has to do with preparing dinner, how we look, what we weigh, how many times we made it to exercise class last week or anything else, comparing ourselves to others is pointless because no two people have the same life, background, and genetics. Especially with all the happy-looking people and delicious-looking healthful meals plastered all over social media, it's easy to fall into this trap. If you see that others are succeeding where you have not, it might be helpful to look at the strategies that they have in place. Perhaps you can mimic or tweak these strategies to achieve your goal.

    Social comparisons can also lead you to believe that you are doing better than you really are. For example, you may think that it's quite acceptable to drink a liter of regular soda daily because your brother polishes off a 2-liter bottle every day. Or you may think that playing basketball once a week is adequate exercise because no one else in your family does that much activity.

9. *Mind reading.* "I ate dessert at my friend's house because I didn't want to hurt her feelings."

    You can't really know what someone else will think. It's better to politely assert your needs.

10. *Magical thinking.* "I'm giving up this list of foods because I think this is the answer to my weight problem."

> I've known people to try one bad diet plan after another because someone told them it would work. Weight management (and physical fitness) require hard work. While tempting, restrictive diets typically lead only to temporary weight loss and are rarely nutritious. For many people, these diets are discouraging and lead to a cycle of restriction and indulgence. There are no magic plans out there. If there were, nearly everyone would be thin and physically fit.

Listen for the "Can't"

Few things are more negative than the word "can't." Often I hear people say things like, "I *can't* eat in that restaurant." What they really mean is that they *choose* not to eat in that restaurant because there are few menu items that fit with their goals. Someone else might say, "I *can't* have cookies in the house because I *can't* control my eating." It's more accurate to say, "I *choose* not to have cookies in the house because I *haven't yet* learned to control my eating." Listen for the "can't," and deliberately choose more empowering language.

Learn To Stop Emotional Eating

Yes, this is something that can be learned. Working on stopping negative thoughts and unhelpful mind traps and deliberately using empowering language can help you in your quest to stop emotional eating. But reaching for food to manage emotions can be a very hard habit to break. Often, a psychotherapist skilled in working with people with disordered eating is the ideal person to help you. Ask your health care provider for a referral if you think a psychotherapist can help you.

Both psychology and biology are at play in emotional eating. People frequently reach for foods they associate with good feelings, such as Mom's cookies or a cheesy casserole. Additionally, stress hormones may crank up appetite, which leads to eating, and the brain's feel-good chemicals respond happily, although temporarily, to the food. Here are a few techniques that may help you learn to break free of emotional eating.

- *Keep a log.* Record your food intake for a week or two. Track what you're eating along with your mood. This process may help you find choice points from which you can learn to change your thinking and behavior and that can teach you to identify your breaking points long before you break. Use the Food Record in Appendix B on page 273 or adapt it for your own needs. Consider keeping a photo log. If you're about to eat, snap a picture. Do this for a week to see in color the choices you've been making.
- *Notice and label your emotions.* Having negative emotions isn't usually bad. Having negative emotions is actually normal. But taking a deep dive into a bag of salty, crunchy snacks because of negative emotions is unhelpful in the long run. Practice noticing and labeling your emotions. Are you sad, anxious, lonely, or mad? Naming them and observing them without judgment will help you learn about them. Many people find that journaling about their emotions is helpful.
- *Imagine handling emotional situations.* In your mind, practice responding to common triggers in ways that don't lead you to overeating. Think about what you can do next time you feel overwhelmed with household chores or the next time you argue with your spouse or whatever situation leads you to eat emotionally. Over and over in your mind, practice acting in desirable ways. Here again, many people find journaling enlightening and empowering.

PREDIABETES: A COMPLETE GUIDE

- *Create a plan.* After imagining responding in positive ways, create a plan for difficult situations. If you need distractions, gather things to help you such as puzzle books, adult coloring books, nail polish, a list of people to call, or a list of activities such as soaking in a bath or playing with your dog. If you know that exercise or meditation helps you cope with strong emotions, plan to take at least 5 minutes for meditation or exercise. You may need more than one plan to address various situations.

- *Practice non-food coping skills.* Regularly soothe yourself without calories. Every day, take time for soothing enjoyment, so when the time comes, you have an arsenal of coping strategies at the ready. I regularly play with Benny, a perpetual puppy. I also call and text my daughters, spend quiet time drinking tea or coffee with my husband, take 5-minute breaks outside, and sit alone sipping a warm and fragrant tea from a beautiful cup. Other people take deep-breathing breaks, use adult coloring books, write in a journal, listen to soothing or uplifting music, chat with a friend, buy themselves flowers, or soak in hot tub. How you choose to soothe yourself is as individual as you are.

    Additionally, a morning ritual potentially has the power to affect your entire day. A ritual is different from a routine in that a ritual holds a deeper meaning. A few examples follow:
    - Express gratitude in thoughts, a journal, or aloud.
    - Reaffirm your goals in writing or aloud.
    - Practice yoga, meditation, or prayer.
    - Watch a sunrise.
    - Visualize good things happening in your day.
    - Recite affirmations or a mantra.

- *Build in food treats.* Whatever food you reach for in times of stress probably has some special meaning to you. Is it chocolate, macaroni and cheese, pizza, or hot-from-the-oven cookies? Whatever it is, be sure to have some now and then. Not as a reward, but simply because you like the way it tastes. Practice enjoying this favorite food in a reasonable amount, perhaps as part of a balanced meal. Simply removing a food's taboo label can be helpful. In this way, you are learning that it's okay to treat yourself and removing the notion of treats as cheats. We all deserve treats, but cheat days are the wrong mindset.

- *Review your personal wellness vision often.* You identified what really matters to you when you created your vision of good health. Regularly look over your personal wellness vision. It's easy to forget what really matters when you're under stress or running in crisis mode. But knowing— and remembering—what's really important steers you to appropriate actions.

Be Consistent

Strive to be at least 80% "perfect," 100% of the time.

Practice Eating Mindfully

Try to describe in great detail the last meal you ate. Draw on memories of all of your senses. Can you describe the colors, textures, and aromas? What can you say about the temperature and the ways in which the food changed as you chewed it? How did eating make you feel both physically and emotionally? Unless you ate very mindfully, you will probably struggle with this exercise.

Mindfulness means paying close attention on purpose and without judgment. Eating mindfully is important in your lifestyle reset because you will gain insight into your body's fullness and hunger cues. You will learn to trust your own wisdom and silence your harsh inner critic. By being fully aware of all that your food gives you, you will likely be satisfied with less food. I try an experiment in my office now and then. I give a small wrapped chocolate to clients and ask them to eat it quickly. Then I give them another one and ask them to eat it very mindfully. Try this simple exercise at home to see what you can learn. Before unwrapping the second piece of chocolate, think about what you expect from it. Ask yourself if this candy has any special meaning to you. Is it something you share with a dear friend or family member? Is it seasonal? Is it a very favorite, or just a candy that you enjoy? Now open it and look at its shape, color, and texture. What does it feel like in your hand? Notice the aroma. What tastes and feelings do you anticipate? Do you notice your mouth watering or your digestive tract moving? Put the chocolate in your mouth and move it around with your tongue. What do you notice now? Slowly bite into it. Notice its texture again. How does the temperature of the chocolate change? Savor the flavor. Once you've swallowed the second piece of candy, think about your experience. How did it compare to the experience of eating the first piece quickly? Answer each of these questions from a scientist's viewpoint. There's no judgment here, just a story to tell.

As you learn to eat more mindfully, you'll become aware of your habitual actions and thoughts. And with this awareness, you can intervene when necessary because you will be able to identify choice points. Mindfulness will help you make food and eating choices based on your preferences, hunger, nutritional needs, and unique experiences and goals. If you enjoy food and look forward to eating, doesn't it make more sense to slow down to enjoy your food than to race through a meal or eat it while driving?

In a world of sensory overload with a constant stream of noise and interruptions, eating mindfully—or doing anything mindfully—is challenging. We've got to deal with kids, bosses, phones ringing, dogs barking, emails, and more! But like so many other parts of your reset, practice gets results, and the payoffs are large.

Be Empowered

- Visit the library to learn about mindful eating and emotional eating. Pick up a book written by an expert such as *End Emotional Eating* by Jennifer L. Taitz, PsyD, or one of several books by mindful eating expert Susan Albers, PsyD.
- Pick at least three meals this week to practice eating mindfully.
- In your mind, run through your day to look for your negative self-talk or any of the common mind traps. Imagine handling those situations in a more positive way.
- As you catch yourself, practice rephrasing negative self-talk.
- Experiment with a morning ritual.
- Create a list of at least five non-food soothing activities.

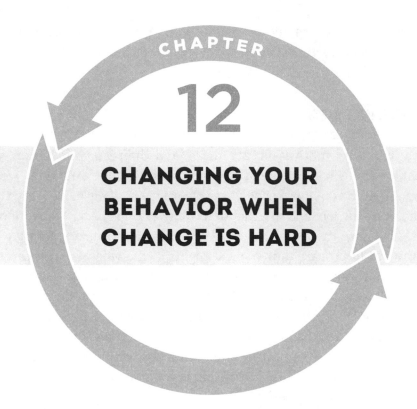

12

CHANGING YOUR BEHAVIOR WHEN CHANGE IS HARD

*I*f healthful lifestyle habits were easy to achieve and maintain, most people—not a mere 24% of the population—would eat the recommended servings of fruit every day. Vegetables would fill most plates. The majority of gym memberships would actually be used. And few people would be chronically sleep deprived and relying on a coffee jolt to get through the day. If there was a quick and lasting fix for weight problems, very few people would be overweight. But the truth is, losing weight and keeping lost pounds off is very, very hard. It's easy to drop an exercise routine and stay up too late to unwind or finish chores. Eating healthfully in a world of unhealthful choices is exceptionally difficult. Throughout this book, you've learned about strategies to set goals and overcome obstacles. We've covered forming and breaking habits and identifying and moving beyond common mind traps. In this chapter, we'll cover additional strategies for behavior change. First and foremost, you should be reassured that behavior change is hard because it's hard, not because of any character flaws.

Finding Motivation

What is it with motivation? It's there, and then it's gone. Often, we think we can will it to come back. But no, it's still gone. And then, we're complimented on how we look or we learn we're going to have a grand-child or a new job, and just like that, motivation is back. Motivation is fickle because there is a cost to every change we make. You may be motivated to prepare dinner most nights of the week, so you can eat more healthfully. But preparing dinner costs you time for something else you'd like to do. You may be motivated to de-stress at yoga class, but the class may be expensive and perhaps going to yoga means that someone else will have to pick up your children at school. We are at risk of reverting to old, unhealthful behaviors when motivation drops. So what can you do if simply wishing to be motivated doesn't help?

Take a First Step

There is power is in doing something even if that something is not your ultimate goal. If you wish you were motivated to get back to your 30-minute afternoon walks, for example, don't wait until the time is just perfect. Instead take a 5-minute walk today or right now. Success breeds success, so give yourself a chance to be successful.

Gather Motivating Items

I have clients who tear out motivating magazine articles, post photos reminding them of their values (such a pictures of grandchildren or a spot in the woods where they like to hike), collect inspiring quotations, and journal about their wishes and dreams. Another client regularly updates a computer document with motivating and inspiring thoughts. These are smart reminders of why we want to make lifestyle changes. Going back to these collections when motivation fizzles is a wonderful way to nurture it back up.

Have a Conversation

Have this conversation either with yourself or with someone you trust. Discuss why you want to change, why you're hesitant to change, how changing will affect other people in good or bad ways, what your obstacles are to changing, and what are reasonable first steps. This is a good time to review Chapter 2 with a careful look at SMART goals, the HURDLE method to overcoming obstacles, and your personal wellness vision. You may even have new things to add to your personal wellness vision.

Use a Pro/Con Chart

As I noted above, there are always good reasons to change and good reasons not to change. Listing them on paper is helpful. Make lists of reasons to change and reasons not to, as in the examples below. It doesn't matter if one list is longer than the other. The length of the lists is rarely important. What matters is the significance of the content. You may find only one con in a long list of cons that is a true obstacle. Moving forward will require you to put your energies into overcoming that one hurdle. Or there may be many obstacles that need your attention. Additionally, you may stumble across one or more reasons to change that are enough to help you get started or stay energized. Feel free to create a pro/con chart for an overarching goal, such as changing your diet, or for a narrow goal, such as packing your lunch. One of my clients is working on a pro/con chart for getting to bed on time. Make a separate chart for each behavior you struggle to change. Don't rush through this exercise. My clients have discovered very interesting things about themselves and their situations. For example, one woman was fearful of losing weight because she didn't know how to handle the unwanted attention of men.

Change or Stay the Same: A Pro/Con Balance Tool

Pros If I change my diet . . .	Cons If I change my diet . . .
I'll lose weight.	Planning my meals will take up time.
I'll be able to wear more fashionable clothing.	I'll have to cook more, which takes up time and energy.
I'll feel so proud of myself.	My family might be unhappy if I stop buying and preparing sweets and fried foods.
I'll worry much less about my health.	I'll have to stop eating at my favorite lunch places every day.
My family will worry less about my health.	I'll worry about regaining weight.
I'll have a good chance of preventing type 2 diabetes.	I'm afraid that I'll get obsessed with the scale.
I might be able to reduce my blood pressure medications and stay off of cholesterol-lowering medications.	I'm afraid that my sister will get jealous and try to sabotage my efforts.
I'll have a good chance of preventing other chronic health problems.	I might get bored with my diet.
I'll have less heartburn and I might get off my heartburn medicine.	It might cost more money.
I'll be a good role model to my family.	
I won't feel guilty or remorseful for eating desserts because they will be occasional treats or small amounts.	
I'll have more energy.	
I'll stop feeling nervous about going to the doctor.	

Change or Stay the Same: A Pro/Con Balance Tool

Pros If I pack my lunch for work . . .	Cons If I pack my lunch for work . . .
I'll eat more nutritious food.	I'll have to grocery shop regularly.
I'm more likely to reach my health goals.	It takes time to pack lunch.
I can save money by not eating out.	I might get bored with my food.
I can save a lot of calories to lose weight.	I won't get to go out with my work buddies.
	Packing a healthful lunch is like announcing that I'm on a diet, and I don't want people to comment about that.

After exploring your reasons to change and to stay the same, identify which list makes the more compelling argument. Do you have stronger reasons to change or to stay exactly where you are? If reviewing these lists doesn't push you forward, ask yourself which items on your cons list are your biggest obstacles. How can you overcome them? Review the HURDLE method. Brainstorm as many options as possible, including thinking-out-of-the-box solutions. If money isn't your concern, but time is, perhaps you could hire someone to help around the house to free up your time for meal planning and preparation. Or you can delegate chores to family members. Can you move forward by taking cooking lessons, getting an accountability partner, working through relationship problems, or making bedtime a few minutes earlier? There are likely many possible solutions once you examine your unique situation and identify what's holding you back. There's a template in Appendix B on page 282 to get you started.

Revisit the Importance, Motivation, and Confidence Ruler

If you've carefully crafted a SMART goal, but haven't been successful, it's a good time to run it through the Importance, Motivation, and Confidence Rulers that we first discussed in Chapter 2.

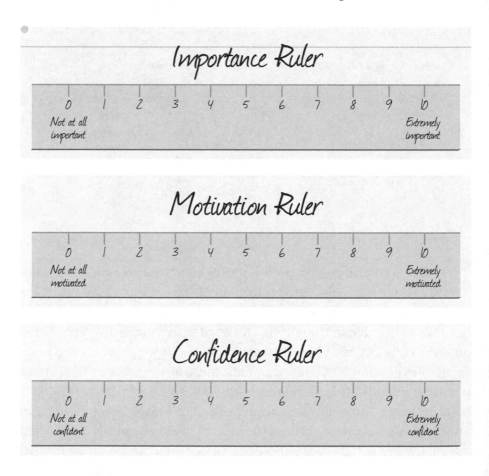

- On a scale of 1–10, how important is this goal to me?
- On a scale of 1–10, how motivated am I to work on this goal?
- One a scale of 1–10, how confident am I that with the resources I have available, I can be reasonably successful with this goal?

If you aren't able to answer each question with at least a 7, either rewrite your goal or put some new strategies in place to boost your confidence. Don't give up. Just keep reworking the goal and/or the plan until you get it in the right place. It's okay to take baby steps. Just keep stepping.

Notice Your Progress

Your progress shows up in a number of ways. It may be a 5-pound weight loss, a lower A1C level, or a reduction in your blood pressure medication. It might be feeling more energized, sleeping more soundly, or noticing that you now exercise regularly and actually look forward to it. Your progress might be related to planning your meals, avoiding greasy food, having less knee pain, climbing the stairs with ease, or no longer feeling terrible remorse when you eat something unplanned. Recognizing your progress and giving yourself a "high five" is both fun and motivating. Use the Progress Report on page 283 in Appendix B to list your accomplishments—those things that have fundamentally changed for you. Review it and add to it often. Share it with people who support your efforts. It may seem silly, unnecessary, and even like bragging, but try keeping up with this list anyway. One day, when your motivation is failing you or you feel that you're not successful with your lifestyle reset, you'll gain so much from reflecting on your progress report.

Notice Today's Non-Scale Victories

You may have already heard of non-scale victories. Although not measured in ounces and pounds, these are things that occurred today that you can feel good about. What behaviors did you engage in today that took you a lot closer to achieving your personal vision of wellness? Unfortunately, too many people put so much emphasis on losing weight that they lose sight that their overall goal is better health and wellness. Or they foolishly expect to follow their diet, exercise, and other lifestyle plans perfectly, noticing only when they mess up and failing to acknowledge what they are doing well. Yes, your weight is important, but it is not everything—not even close. Think about what you did well today in your efforts to take care of your health. Jot down these little (or big) triumphs in your journal, on your calendar, or on the Daily Victories Report on page 284 in Appendix B. Include the time you passed up on the supermarket samples, took a few deep breaths to calm yourself instead of reaching for food, caught yourself eating too fast and then slowed down, or squeezed a 10-minute walk into your busy day. Reflecting on your day in this way is a wonderful reminder to slow down and appreciate the difficulty of a lifestyle reset and to appreciate both your efforts and your successes, no matter the size.

The difference between the Progress Report and the Daily Victories Report can be confusing. Use the Progress Report to list new habits and health improvements—things that identify your overall progress. List daily accomplishments on the Daily Victories Report. The overall goal of the Daily Victories Report is to take excess focus off of things you could have done better and to help you take note of the little things you did well.

Make Healthy the Easy Choice

Because lasting change is hard to make, it's smart to set up your home, office, car, and other parts of your usual environment in ways that facilitate, instead of hinder, wholesome eating and living. For example, keeping cookies on your kitchen counter is more hazardous to your health than storing them in a hard-to-reach cabinet. Similarly, you're more likely to meet your fruit goal if you put a bowl of apples on your counter or cut-up melon in your refrigerator than you are if the apples are hidden and the melon is uncut. Wearing comfortable shoes may prompt you to take an after-lunch walk, and putting the treadmill and TV in the same room may

246

help you get in a few extra minutes of exercise here and there. These are examples of simple strategies that can help you make the better choice. With some creative thought, you can surely come up with many more strategies to help ensure long-term success. After all, motivation comes and goes; willpower is hugely overestimated and unreliable; and the environment, with an abundance of food and too many opportunities to be physically inactive, is stacked against us. Proactively setting up your environment reduces your minute-to-minute efforts.

Think about those cookies on the kitchen counter. If you are spending time in the evening fighting with yourself about whether to eat them and how many to eat, or if you are bargaining a cookie for an extra 10 minutes of exercise, you are wearing down your emotional energy. Put those cookies away, so you can save your energy for things you have less control over. Here are several strategies that have helped my clients and me.

- If you have unhealthful, tempting food at home, keep it behind closed cabinets, in opaque containers, or both. Use this out-of-sight, out-of-mind technique often—at home, at work, in the car, everywhere.
- Pre-portion washed and ready-to-eat fruits and veggies into small containers or baggies. Make grabbing a bag of fresh produce as easy as grabbing a bag of chips.
- Pre-portion chips and crackers into small baggies, so you get just the right amount each time. Your brain won't have to think so much when you pack lunch or reach for a snack.
- Serve meats and starches from the stove, but take fruits and vegetables to the table. This step should encourage you to skip second helpings of some foods, but not others.
- Go out of your way to avoid temptation. Clients have switched gas stations to keep themselves from buying a hot dog or coffee and pastry with every fill-up. Others drive a different route to bypass a particularly enticing takeout place.

- Pack healthful work snacks every Monday. If you snack at work, be sure you have good choices. Take five pieces of fruit or other wholesome snacks each Monday to eat all week long.
- Eat from small dishes. A small serving looks bigger on an 8- or 9-inch plate than it does on an 11-inch plate. Treat yourself to small, attractive cereal bowls and even smaller dessert bowls.
- Instead of candy in a candy dish, fill your bowl with decorative stones or marbles. Or say goodbye to the dish and create a welcoming spot with photographs, flowers, or art.
- Keep a pair of comfortable shoes nearby to allow yourself a walking break.
- De-clutter some space in your home for some indoor exercise. You'll need it when the weather turns bad.

Stay Out of Food Jail

Over the years, many clients have told me they have been in food jail—that awful, painful place where they are forced to eat food that doesn't interest them, where they are not allowed to eat what they really want, where they are often hungry, and where they feel they have no control over their food choices.

Diet books and programs are popular, in part, because of their clear and strict rules. Dieters know what to eat, when to eat, how to eat, and what not to eat. There is security in knowing exactly what to do. However, unless you wrote that book yourself, the rules and lists of good and bad foods probably don't fit your life and preferences very well. Even if you wrote the diet plan and you gave yourself a bunch of strict rules, you would probably eventually find yourself in food jail clamoring to break out. This is such a common situation. A dieter is happy following a boring, strict diet because weight is coming off or blood glucose or cholesterol levels have improved. The long list of rules leaves little room for making a mistake. So what's the problem? Eventually, strict dieters hate food rules and food jail so much that they quit the plan. They frequently swing all the way to the other end of the dieting spectrum and eat with abandon, as if they might be hit by a bus tomorrow. Their labs don't look so good anymore. They gain the weight back, feel guilt or shame, revert to old habits, and set themselves up for more on-and-off dieting.

You can avoid food jail and make your lifestyle habits stick by saying a very loud "no" to restrictive diets and draconian food rules. You can also use flexible food rules appropriately to keep yourself on plan without too much mental arguing going on.

There are three parts to making food rules work for you instead of against you.

1. *Create rules to help you make the right choices most of the time.* These are rules that you like, and they help you make good decisions. They are unique to your life, your routines, and your food preferences. A few of my food rules (and one exercise rule) follow:
   - I eat three meals every day.
   - At dinner, I eat more vegetables than any other type of food.
   - Whenever I eat pizza, I eat a bowl of salad before my first slice of pizza and a second bowl of salad before my second slice of pizza.
   - I don't eat after dinner.
   - I don't eat sweets in the morning.
   - I don't eat food that others bring into my office.
   - I exercise every morning before work.

   You may or may not like my rules and that's okay. They're for me. I like them. I never feel deprived by them, and I never have to decide to exercise in the morning or whether or not dip into the candy jar at work. I don't have to think about it. I don't argue with myself. I just know what to do.

2. *Create exceptions to your rules.* These exceptions need to be created in advance and not on the fly. An important purpose of food rules is to free you of an internal argument of should

I or shouldn't I. Making exceptions on the fly is the same as breaking your rules, and this usually comes after one of those tiresome mental arguments. Here are two examples of mine.

- I don't eat food brought into my office *except* when it's a healthful lunch in place of my own healthful lunch or *except* when the food is so unusual that it's my only opportunity to experience it (such as a home-prepared item from a coworker's unique culture).
- I don't eat after dinner *except* when dinner was so early or so small that I'm hungry.

Just as your rules are unique, your exceptions must also be unique. Otherwise, they just won't fit your life. You may realize that you consume a few hundred calories tasting supermarket or big box store samples each week, suggesting that you will benefit from a rule around this. Your rule with exceptions may look like this: I don't eat grocery store samples *except* when it's only a fruit or vegetable or *except* when it will help me decide if I should buy the product.

3. *Reevaluate your rules and exceptions periodically.* Continue to create new rules and tweak old ones. Remember, these are rules to keep you on track but also to keep you out of food jail. If they start to feel like jail, something needs to change. Your ultimate goal has got to be sustainable lifestyle changes, not moving back and forth between rigid diet and lifestyle plans and an anything-goes kind of routine.

Halt an Impending Relapse

Even though we are approaching your lifestyle reset in such a way to make it sustainable, relapses are still possible. You can guard against a full-blown relapse by protecting your new habits and attitude. Recognize *all* the little changes you've made that add up to something bigger—better health and wellness. Pat yourself on the back, and soldier on. Maintain your Progress Report and your Daily Victories Report. Keep looking for obstacles and make plans to overcome them. How will you handle food at a party or on vacation? How will you get exercise when the weather is bad or when your schedule changes? Form the habit of scanning your day and week ahead for potential roadblocks and use the HURDLE method to find workable solutions.

Shake off little lapses. We all have them. Note them for what they are—little lapses that won't have a big impact if they are few and far between. Many little lapses, however, are a warning sign that a relapse is in the making. Try to identify these problem behaviors and thoughts before they take hold and drag you in a downward spiral. Look for these red flags.

- You're eating more junk food or drinking more alcohol than usual.
- You're sick of your food choices.
- You're sneaking food.
- Your intake of fruits and vegetables has dropped significantly.
- You've been skipping meals.
- You're eating out more often than usual.
- You've stopped weighing yourself because you don't want to see the number.
- You feel like you're in food jail.
- You feel depressed or guilty about your health or your health habits.
- You're relying on coffee or another caffeine source to keep you going.
- You noticed that you've been rushing through your meals and not listening to your hunger cues.
- If you had been recording your food intake, you've stopped or have been tracking your intake only sporadically.
- You've put off appointments with your health care providers because you don't want to discuss difficult things.

- You've not been regular with your exercise routine.
- You welcome excuses to eat unhealthfully or skip exercise instead of finding solutions to obstacles.
- You hate your exercise routine.
- You've been staying up too late.
- You can't identify things in your day that help you manage stress.
- You find yourself "catastrophyzing" or engaging in negative self-talk without reframing.
- You didn't stick to your plan, so you decide to "blow it" even more and start fresh tomorrow.

As soon as you notice these warning signs or red flags, seek help from a coach or a friend, analyze your situation and make a plan to get back on track, set new goals, review your personal wellness vision, find new motivators, or use any strategy that you find helpful. Don't panic or give in to negative thinking. Stay true to your ultimate goal to form new lifestyle habits rather than cycle between restrictive plans and a free-for-all.

Be Empowered

- Start or add to your Progress Report.
- Start or add to your Daily Victories Report.
- Share your progress and daily victories on social media, using #LifestyleReset and @NutritionJill.
- Review your personal wellness vision and most recent set of 3-month goals.
- Set new 3-month or weekly goals if appropriate.

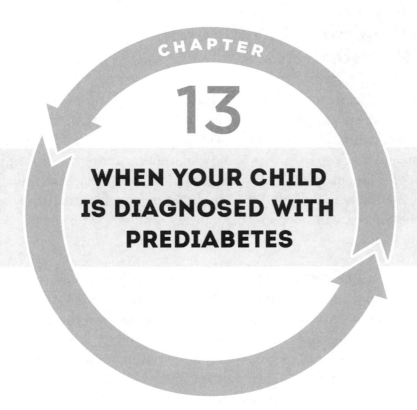

CHAPTER
13

WHEN YOUR CHILD IS DIAGNOSED WITH PREDIABETES

As adults, a diagnosis of prediabetes is likely to evoke some emotion. We might feel fear, worry, or guilt when we learn of this diagnosis. But when it's our child who has prediabetes, putting him or her at risk for type 2 diabetes, it's likely that our own emotions are magnified. You may feel panic, guilt, or a heightened sense of urgency. While it is urgent to address your child's health, keep in mind that even among children and teens with prediabetes, a diagnosis of type 2 diabetes is not inevitable. With careful attention, you, your child, and your child's health care provider can work to manage this health problem.

14 Steps to Help Your Child with Prediabetes

The risk factors for prediabetes and type 2 diabetes are similar for both children and adults. Likewise, the same healthy lifestyle habits discussed throughout this book will help your child, too. Here's a bit more guidance specific to helping children. In this chapter, as in the rest of this book, prediabetes refers to pre–type 2 diabetes. Although you are likely to find insight in this chapter if your child has type 1 diabetes, you will need to work closely with a team of health care professionals.

1. *Ask your child's health care provider if your child is overweight.* Although overweight and obesity increase the risk of developing prediabetes and type 2 diabetes, not everyone with these diagnoses is overweight. If your child is overweight, ask if the appropriate goal is to maintain weight during growth, slow the rate of weight gain, or to lose weight. Whether or not weight loss is a good idea for a child has to do with several things, including the child's age, height, and weight.

2. *Ask for a referral.* Once your child's health care provider has explained the diagnosis and made some basic recommendations, ask for a referral to a registered dietitian or a registered dietitian nutritionist (RD or RDN). This is the person to help you and other members of your family plan healthful meals and snacks. A skilled RDN will help you and your child set reasonable, actionable goals to help the entire family feel empowered and be successful.

3. *Make it a family affair.* Even if only one member of the family has health concerns, it's important for the entire family to live healthfully. This scenario supports your child and helps to prevent him or her from feeling isolated or stigmatized. Besides, there's no member of the family who doesn't need to eat and live healthfully.

4. *Avoid negative language.* Take another look at Chapter 11. Just as it's harmful for you to use negative language when talking about yourself, using negative language is hurtful to your child. Avoid saying things like, "You can't have chips and cookies." Try rephrasing the language to something more positive like, "Let's pick out a couple types of fruit for your lunch this week and leave the cookies for a special occasion."

5. *Give your child choices.* If you've made it a goal for your family to eat dessert only three times per week, for example, allow your child to choose what or when. You might give your kids the choice of having an ice cream sandwich at the beach this afternoon or waiting until after dinner for a small cupcake.

6. *Be supportive, not controlling.* Ask your child about changes he or she wants to make. This gives your child an important sense of control. Provide a supportive environment—one without judgment and stigma. Provide healthful food and drink without excessive temptation of unhealthful food choices. Avoid telling your child when he or she has eaten enough. Instead allow your child to learn about individual hunger cues. Provide plenty of opportunities to be active.

7. *Make activity fun.* Your children may enjoy team sports, martial arts, ballet, or running. As a family, you might like biking, hiking, and swimming. Maybe you can purchase an active game for your gaming console. Whatever you do, focus on fun activities and not punishing activities. Don't talk about exercise as punishment for eating too much or being overweight. As you read in Chapter 8, exercise has plenty of rewards. And, besides, having a health concern is not a reason to be punished.

8. *Model good eating and exercise behaviors.* Kids definitely pick up both behaviors and values from their parents. Show them

that you value good health by eating wholesome foods and being physically active.

9. *Eat more meals at home.* And eat them together. Eat at a table, not on the couch while watching TV. If time is tight, here are some tips:
   - Plan fast and simple meals like soup and sandwiches.
   - Combine prepared foods like rotisserie chicken with scratch items like brown rice and broccoli.
   - Bring out your slow cooker to have dinner ready when you are.

10. *Include your kids in the meal planning and prep.* Dole out tasks that are appropriate for age. Young children can set the table, rinse fruit, and count the proper number of carrots for a recipe. Older children can cut vegetables and use the stove. Make it fun by allowing children to pick recipes or themes. Try out taco night or throw a blanket on the floor and pretend it's an outdoor picnic.

11. *Eliminate—or severely limit—sugar-sweetened beverages.* Sugary sodas, teas, fruit drinks, and sports drinks provide a lot of calories and a lot of added sugar. Yet they offer little in the way of nutrition. If you do have them, make them a rarity and keep the serving to approximately 1 cup.

12. *Don't use food to reward or punish.* This tactic can have lasting effects, making it hard for your child to have a healthy relationship with food.

13. *Enforce a bedtime.* Because kids have plenty of activities and homework, getting to bed on time is a challenge. Yet it's critical for good health and good decision-making.

14. *Be patient.* It's hard for us to make lasting changes. It's hard for our kids, too, especially when they are faced with unhealthful messages in the media and from friends and when there is such an abundance of eating opportunities. Don't expect perfection. Simply look for opportunities to make smart choices and to teach your children how to make smart choices.

Be Empowered

- Seek advice from your child's health care provider. Ask for a referral to a registered dietitian nutritionist.
- Pick two to five changes to implement. If appropriate, do this collaboratively with your child and other family members.
- Once you and your family have mastered these initial goals, create a few more.

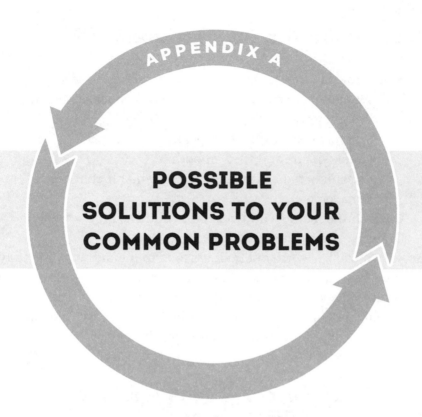

POSSIBLE SOLUTIONS TO YOUR COMMON PROBLEMS

In Chapter 2, we reviewed the HURDLE method to overcoming obstacles. A template to help you work through the six steps is on page 270. Often, the best solutions to problems are the ones you figure out on your own. At the same time, it's helpful to have someone brainstorm some ideas with you. The following pages will help you with your brainstorming sessions for various common obstacles when you don't have someone to help you or you prefer not to involve others. Just use the following as suggestions. These ideas, which came from my years of experience and from my clients, are likely no better than your own ideas.

When You're Too Busy for Breakfast

- Find a few favorite grab-and-go options such as these:
  - Whole-wheat tortilla with reduced-fat cheese heated in the microwave
  - Whole-wheat waffle with peanut butter
  - Greek yogurt and fruit smoothie
  - Overnight oats with strawberries and blueberries
  - Tuna sandwich
- Cook oatmeal or egg and vegetable muffins on the weekend. Grab a single serving each morning.
- Take a week's worth of breakfast food to the office on Monday. Prepare and eat your breakfast at work. A few good choices are cottage cheese with fruit and muesli, yogurt with fruit and dry cereal, and an English muffin with almond butter and banana.
- Ask a family member to prepare your breakfast.

When Your Partner "Won't Eat That" and Doesn't Offer Support

I've heard this a lot from clients. My client wants to eat healthfully, but his or her spouse or partner doesn't like wholesome food or feels punished when trigger foods are removed from the house. Because our worlds operate more smoothly when we are in sync with those important to us, it's worth starting an honest discussion. Maybe not so surprisingly, sometimes a partner is less than enthused about a diet change because it feels threatening. I've known of people who don't want their spouses to lose weight because it might make them more attractive to others. And I've known of people who sabotage their partners' weight loss efforts because it makes them feel guilty for not changing their own diets.

And sometimes people have no idea that they're being hurtful. It's not fair to guess someone else's motives, but it's smart to start the conversation. Instead of asking your partner to be more supportive, it's helpful to give specific suggestions, such as asking him or her to be open to eating meatless meals twice a week, keeping your favorite cookies out of the house, not offering you ice cream every night after dinner, or picking up a chore to give you a chance to take a walk. You may not get everything that you feel you need, but having this honest conversation will likely get you more than if you continue to seethe because you have little support or give up because that's simpler.

When There's Too Much Tempting Food at Work

- Create a rule with exceptions. Review this section on page 249 in Chapter 12. My own simple rule is that I do not eat office junk food unless it is so unusual that I'll miss a unique experience. I had a rule for 8 years in a different office that I dipped into the candy jar only on Wednesdays. I always had Wednesday to look forward to, and I never argued with myself on the other days.
- Ask officemates to keep tempting foods in only one spot. Try to avoid that one spot.
- Ask coworkers if they also want to eliminate certain types of food from work. You might be pleasantly surprised. After all, you aren't the only one who cares about what you eat.
- Pack your coffee in a thermal container, so you can avoid the junk food in the office kitchen when you need a coffee refill.

When You're at a Party

Success starts with intention, so avoid the temptation to simply wing it. Also resist the temptation to avoid parties because you fear them. Becoming socially isolated is no good solution.

- Determine your tradeoffs. Will you skip appetizers and starchy sides to enjoy a piece of birthday cake, or do you prefer a cocktail and an appetizer? It helps to make decisions before heading out the door.
- Be cautious with alcohol. It has a way of leading people to greater food temptations. Start with a low-calorie, nonalcoholic drink and have a second nonalcoholic beverage after you drink a cocktail or glass of wine.
- Take the edge off your hunger before going to the party, if appropriate. There is usually no reason to pre-eat, which often results in eating too much overall. But if you feel uncomfortably hungry when you're teased with an abundance of party food, you will likely find it hard to hold control. It's okay to enter a party with a normal appetite, but if you need a small snack first, choose something healthful and filling like an apple, an orange, or a glass of vegetable juice. At the party, take your first bites of lower-calorie foods like fresh fruits and veggies or steamed shrimp.
- Be active. If dancing or playing games is part of the party, join in.
- If appropriate, bring a healthful dish to share.
- Keep yourself occupied with conversation and other non-food activities.
- When you've had enough to eat, position yourself far from the food.
- Remind yourself that just because you've always indulged in party food, doesn't mean that you can't change that.

When You're on Vacation

Again, success starts with the intention of being successful. Avoid the mentality that you deserve unhealthful eating because you're on vacation. Really, no one deserves unhealthful eating. Everyone deserves to eat healthfully, and everyone deserves just a bit of not-so-nutritious food tossed into the mix for a little extra fun.

- Pack food for the trip.
    - If you are traveling by car, use a cooler and fill it with fruit, veggies, yogurt, low-fat cheese and cottage cheese, vegetable juice, hard-boiled eggs, and a turkey or tuna sandwich.
    - Whether you have a cooler or not, you can still carry nuts, dried fruit, some fresh fruits and vegetables, peanut butter, whole-grain crackers, and granola bars or fiber-rich cereal bars.
    - If you are traveling by plane, pack a small amount of perishable food in a plastic bag. Keep it cold with ice in a separate plastic bag. Airport security will probably want you to get rid of the ice before you go through screening. Once you're through security, stop by a food vendor and kindly ask to refill your plastic bag with more ice.
- Once you're at your destination, stock up on additional wholesome options. If you don't have access to a refrigerator, keep a small amount of perishable food fresh with ice and an ice bucket. Or pack a collapsible vinyl cooler in your luggage for use while away.
- Snack only on fruit.
- Ask locals for restaurant ideas and search menus online before going out to eat.
- Opt for a walking tour instead of a bus tour.
- Carry a refillable water bottle.
- Find a local gym.
- Decide in advance what amount of treats is reasonable for you. A glass of wine a day? A couple of desserts over the week? Create your rules and exceptions, so you have a working blueprint to follow.

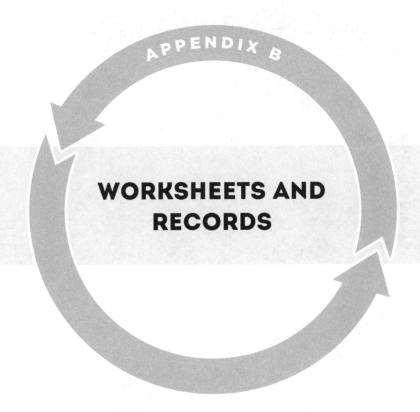

WORKSHEETS AND RECORDS

*F*eel free to make as many copies as necessary of any of the pages in Appendix B. Consider treating yourself to an attractive notebook or journal to gather all of your worksheets and plans together.

- Healthy Me: Personal Wellness Vision
- My 3-Month Behavioral Goals
- SMART Goals Worksheet
- Goal-Tracker
- HURDLE Method to Overcoming Obstacles
- Weight-Tracker
- Food Record

- Detailed Weekly Menu Planner
- Weekly Plate Method Planner
- Mix-and-Match Weekly Menu Planner
- Activity/Inactivity Record
- To Change or Stay the Same: A Pro/Con Balance Tool
- Progress Report
- Daily Victories Report

Healthy Me: Personal Wellness Vision

Hint: Review the tips on page 20. Write in the present tense.

Today's date: _____

When I envision my healthiest self, this is what I see and what I look forward to.

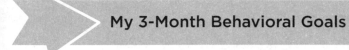

My 3-Month Behavioral Goals

Hint: Review the section on 3-month behavioral goals on page 21. Write in the present tense.

Anticipated completion date: _____

_____

_____

_____

_____

_____

_____

SMART Goals Worksheet

Write your goals in the space provided. Check that it meets each of the five SMART goal principles. Then list any steps you must take to ensure your success (such as get up early, grocery shop, ask for support, etc.).

S: Specific (or Stranger Test): Be specific about what you will do, how you will do it, and where you will do it. If your goal is specific, anyone who reads it will know your plan.

M: Measureable: Can you measure and objectively report your success?

A: Action-Orientated: Your goal must be stated as a behavior. What action will you take?

R: Realistic: With reasonable effort, can you achieve this goal with the resources you have?

T: Timely: When you will do this and when you will assess your results?

Goals:

1) _____

_____

S:_____   M:_____   A:_____   R:_____   T:_____

Additional steps to success: _____

_____

2) _____

_____

S:_____   M:_____   A:_____   R:_____   T:_____

Additional steps to success: _____

_____

3) _____

_____

S:_____   M:_____   A:_____   R:_____   T:_____

Additional steps to success: _____

_____

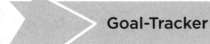

Goal-Tracker

Select as many as five goals, such as eat breakfast, pack lunch, and walk after dinner. Record your progress on a checklist. This process is objective; either you met your goal (ate breakfast, packed lunch, walked after dinner) or you did not. At the end of the week, assess your results. Begin by looking at it from a scientist's perspective. Ask what went well, what didn't, how things could have gone better, what was enjoyable, and what wasn't. Use this information to tweak or change your goals as necessary.

Date: _____

GOAL	Day 1	Day 2	Day 3	Day 4	Day 5	Day 6	Day 7	RESULT

HURDLE Method to Overcoming Obstacles

Obstacles are always lurking. To be successful with your lifestyle reset, get into the habit of looking for and anticipating those obstacles. This worksheet will help you overcome them.

H: How is your upcoming schedule different? Think about your day, week, or month and look at your calendar. What event is unusual or scheduled for an unusual time?

_____

_____

_____

U: Understand how these appointments or obligations could derail you from eating well or exercising, or otherwise get in the way of your goals. Will something prevent you from eating a meal or getting to your exercise class on time? Will someone else be in charge of your meals or your schedule? How might some activity or problem prevent you from sticking to your lifestyle plan?

_____

_____

_____

R: Record your options. Write down every possible solution even if it seems silly.

_____

_____

_____

_____

_____

D: Decide on a solution. From the list above, pick one or more options that are doable and likely to bring you success.

_____

_____

_____

L: List the steps. Record everything you must do to make this solution work. If you must buy something, wake up early, ask for help, or prepare something, write it down.

_____

_____

_____

E: Exercise your choice and **Evaluate** it.

Carry out your plan. How did it go? Would you do it this way again, or make some changes? What did you learn? What will you do differently next time?

_____

_____

_____

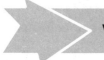

Weight-Tracker

On the chart below, record your weight and total weight loss.

Date	Today's Weight	Total Weight Loss

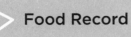

Food Record

Make one copy for each day, or create your own version in your journal or on your computer.

Hint: Review the tips for recording your food intake on page 86. Record everything you eat and drink, or target only your weak areas such as eating out, dinner, snacks, dessert, or other trouble foods, places, or circumstances.

Day: _____   **Date:** _____

Today's goal: _____

Time/Meal (Place)	Food, Amount, Preparation	Notes (mood, hunger level, special circumstances, realizations)

Detailed Weekly Menu Planner

Fill in your plans for each dinner. If desired, do the same for each lunch and breakfast.

Weekly Menu Planner

	MON	TUES	WED	THURS	FRI	SAT	SUN
D							
L							
B							

274

Detailed Weekly Menu Planner: Example

Weekly Menu Planner

	MON	TUES	WED	THURS	FRI	SAT	SUN
D	Salmon with Lemon Basil Sauce Sautéed spinach Cauliflower Couscous Farro	Lentil and Sweet Potato Chili Salad Clementines	Citrus and Herb Chicken Thighs Brown rice Sautéed zucchini and onions	Whole-wheat spaghetti Meat sauce Salad	Homemade pizza Green beans Salad Strawberries	Out to dinner	Veggie and cheese paninis Chunky Gazpacho
L							
B							

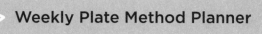

Weekly Plate Method Planner

Use this planner to help you plan balanced dinners with lots of variety and appropriate portions. You can use it for lunch as well, if desired. Review page 52 for a more in-depth look at the Plate Method. Remember to use a 9-inch plate.

Monday		
1/4 Plate Lean Meat or Other Protein	1/4 Plate Grain or Starchy Vegetable	1/2 Plate Nonstarchy Vegetable

Tuesday		
1/4 Plate Lean Meat or Other Protein	1/4 Plate Grain or Starchy Vegetable	1/2 Plate Nonstarchy Vegetable

Wednesday		
1/4 Plate Lean Meat or Other Protein	1/4 Plate Grain or Starchy Vegetable	1/2 Plate Nonstarchy Vegetable

Thursday		
1/4 Plate Lean Meat or Other Protein	1/4 Plate Grain or Starchy Vegetable	1/2 Plate Nonstarchy Vegetable

Friday		
1/4 Plate Lean Meat or Other Protein	1/4 Plate Grain or Starchy Vegetable	1/2 Plate Nonstarchy Vegetable

Saturday		
1/4 Plate Lean Meat or Other Protein	1/4 Plate Grain or Starchy Vegetable	1/2 Plate Nonstarchy Vegetable

Sunday		
1/4 Plate Lean Meat or Other Protein	1/4 Plate Grain or Starchy Vegetable	1/2 Plate Nonstarchy Vegetable

Mix-and-Match Weekly Menu Planner

Fill in the necessary number of entrees, starches, and vegetables. Add additional items, including foods for lunch, if desired.

Entrees	
Starches	
Nonstarchy vegetables	
Other	

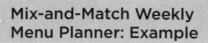

Mix-and-Match Weekly Menu Planner: Example

Entrees	Salmon with Lemon Basil Sauce
	Lentil and Sweet Potato Chili
	Veggie and cheese paninis
	Rotisserie chicken
	Black beans and rice
	Pot roast

Starches	Brown rice
	Quinoa
	Small white potatoes
	Whole-wheat pasta

Nonstarchy vegetables	Fresh broccoli for roasting
	Green beans
	Carrots, celery, and onions
	Riced cauliflower
	At least one more fresh or frozen vegetable
	Salad vegetables for at least 3 nights

Other For lunches	Whole-grain bread
	Yogurt
	Cottage cheese
	Fresh and canned fruit
	Turkey or chicken from the deli
	Raw veggies
	Hummus
	Prepared soup

Activity/Inactivity Record

Record your activities throughout your day. Look for blocks of time in which you are inactive, defined as less than 3 minutes of activity in a 30-minute period. See page 208 for more discussion.

Day: _____   **Date:** _____

Time	Activity	Minutes Active or Standing/Total Minutes

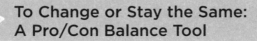

To Change or Stay the Same: A Pro/Con Balance Tool

Under Pros, identify the benefits of changing a specific behavior or achieving a certain goal. Under Cons, list the negative effects of changing the behavior or achieving the goal. Use a second page if necessary. Once done, explore ways to overcome the obstacles you noted in your list of Cons. See page 241 for a detailed discussion of using a Pro/Con sheet.

Pros	Cons
New Behavior:_____	New Behavior:_____

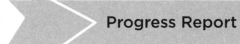

Progress Report

List your accomplishments including better health, improved attitudes, and new, solid behaviors and habits. List them all, and reflect on them regularly. See page 245 for more discussion about your Progress Report.

Date	Accomplishment

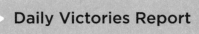

Daily Victories Report

Scan through your day to identify each victory—big and small. List each behavior related to your lifestyle reset that makes you proud. Include positive language and mindset. See page 245 for more discussion about your Daily Victories Report and how it differs from the Progress Report.

Date	Accomplishment

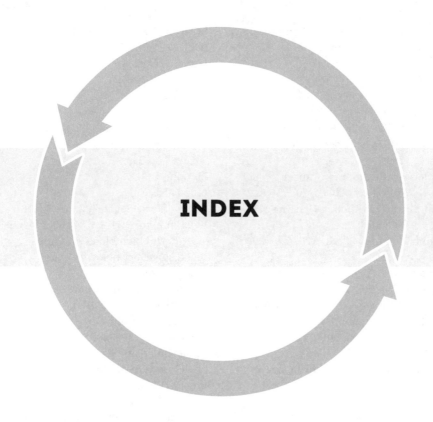

INDEX

Note: Page numbers in **bold** indicate an in-depth discussion. Recipe titles are in *italics*.